MEDICAL TALES

AND STORIES OF HEALING AND

RECOVERY

I0555087

DR. HANI RAOUL KHOUZAM

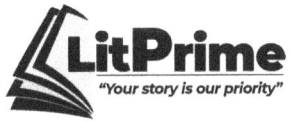

"Your story is our priority"

LitPrime Solutions
21250 Hawthorne Blvd
Suite 500, Torrance, CA 90503
www.litprime.com
Phone: 1-800-981-9893

Published by LitPrime Solutions: 06/07/2024

ISBN: 979-8-88703-370-9(sc)
ISBN: 979-8-88703-371-6(e)

Library of Congress Control Number: 2024911370

Tales and stories are based on true events. The individuals' identity and geographic locations were changed to protect the confidentiality and integrity of patient-doctor therapeutic relationships and the author's professional colleagues and associates.

LitPrime confirmed the described events did not violate any registered copyright ownerships.

In gratitude to my late father, Raoul; my late mother, Jeannette;to my sisters, Hoda and Héla; my brother, Hadi; my wife, Lynn; and my children, Andrew, Adam, Andrea, my son in law Nic and my granddaughters, Abigail and Liliana. Sincere appreciation to my friends, colleagues, teachers, mentors, instructors, and supervisors.

Suffering produces endurance, and endurance produces character, and character produces hope.

Romans 5:3-4.

CONTENTS

* Segments previously published in medical and online publications

TALE I

*Autism Spectrum Disorder**

The Tallest Tree in the Woods of Wisconsin

Atticus had difficulty with verbal communication. He was extremely bothered by noises and sounds. Although he was artistic and could sit for hours drawing amazing rainbow colored figurines. Since birth he could not easily go to sleep. His parents realized that he was different in his appearance and in his demeanors from his 2 older brothers. His dad was optimistic and hopeful that his son will eventually grow out his difficulties. To the contrary his mom was known as being a realist and yearned for Atticus to follow her family heritage of successful entrepreneurs. These dreams where shattered when Atticus was diagnosed with *Autism Spectrum Disorder.*

Not Able to Sleep

Atticus had difficulty falling asleep, with restlessness, interrupted sleep and frequently waking up early. The disturbed sleep patterns had detrimental effects not only on Atticus but on his whole family. Several extensive medical and neurologic evaluations with multiple behavioral and social interventions since he was born could not alleviate the persistent sleep disturbances. As a consequence of the inadequate restful sleep, Atticus experienced complications in his daily functioning which were manifested by aggressive behaviors, prevalent sadness, hyperactivity, irritability, poor learning and the inflection of self-injuries such as scratching his arms and his legs with plastic knives.

At the age of 7 and at the urging of Atticus maternal grandparents, Atticus was enrolled in a Summer camp which specialized in providing recreational activities for children with *Autism Spectrum Disorder.*

What Would Happen in the Summer Camp ?

This particular 12-days Summer camp enrolled male children with *Autism Spectrum Disorder* between the age of 7 and 10 years old. The children participated in various specially designed sport and outdoor activities that were intended to meet their cognitive and behavioral needs. Children were assigned to different groups and each group had 6 children. Each group had coaches manage and supervise the daily schedules of activities, meals time, periods of rest, bedtime and waking up time. Like Atticus many of the children had ongoing sleep disturbances such as difficulty falling asleep, inconsistent sleep, bedtime restlessness, early awakenings and frequent waking up in the middle of the night.

Consistently and repeatedly at bedtime, every night Atticus along with the other children in his group were told a story about a particular tree.

The Tree and its Plight

Once upon a time there was an old tall tree which did not grow any leaves although it was alive and big and was taller than all the other trees in the woods, No birds or squirrels would build their nests on its branches, thinking that it was not a living tree. The tree was sad, lonely and kept wishing that one day some birds or squirrels will use its branches to build their nest and keep her company specially during the cold winter Wisconsin months. One day a squirrel who was lost in the woods and was feeling the cold breeze and instantly realized that he needed to build his own nest before Winter arrives. Looking all around, all the trees were already occupied by nests of birds and squirrels. Noticing the tall tree, it seemed to be a perfect location for building a nest. The tree welcomed the squirrel and pointed many spots on one of its twisted branches to build a secure and sheltered nest. Other squirrels made fun of this plan because they still believed that this tall tree was dead, and it will not survive the Winter storms and with the snow falling, the nest will be destroyed and crashed to the cold frozen grounds. Birds flew over and laughed at the squirrel and mocking the very large nest that was built.

The Homeless Squirrel

The squirrel was very happy with his finished spacious nest and the tree was so glad to have a new company. Climbing on its tallest branches showed a vista of fields that were abundant with acorns. The tree also pointed areas of fallen pecans and walnuts that were not seen by the other squirrels and birds. The squirrel worked hard and gathered so many acorns, walnuts and pecans and stored them in his large nest for the long cold Winter.

Harsh Winter

That Wisconsin Winter came with unusual extremely cold air, frigid winds and many snow storms. The tree with its long strong branches offered an amazing protection for the squirrel nest in addition to providing extra warmth against the blustery cold winds. As the frigid cold days continued with snowflakes turning to ice, the other squirrels and birds' nests that were built on other trees began to fall from the weight of the ice. Their stored food of nuts were scattered and buried under the ice and they were cold frozen, homeless and hungry.

The tall tree was very, very sad to see what was happening to these destitute birds and squirrels and asked her only inhabitant her squirrel if he could invite all the birds and squirrels who lost their nests to come and share his very spacious and large nest. The squirrel came down from the tallest tree and welcomed all the homeless birds and squirrels with their babies to his large nest. He was so happy to shelter them from the harsh Winter weather and to share his abundance of stored food. The tall tree was so joyful to have the company of so many birds, squirrels and their babies. This amazing and unexpected company took away the so many years of lonely and sad living.

Spring Arrived

The cold Winter gradually left to make room for the Spring, the ice melted, and the sun began to shine on other trees with their branches and leaves. The tall tree then started to think that sooner than later she will lose her abundant company of friends who will abandon her to live on other trees with leaves and she will be left once more all alone with so many branches and no leaves. The squirrels and the birds felt the tall tree's sadness and began to wonder on how to help that loving tree in growing leaves on her so many branches. They noticed that in nearby fields, the farmers usually spread a certain type of dark soil on the ground before they water to grow their green crops. They whispered among themselves and found that this soil is full of top soil. So, they carried in their little mouths that dark soil and spread it all around the tall tree. When the rain came, the dark soil disappeared and seemed to be absorbed by the tall free underground roots.

The Tree Growing New Leaves

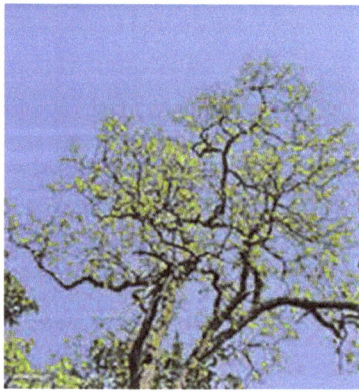

Then miraculously bright green leaves grew all over its many countless branches. The squirrels and birds invited so many other squirrels and birds to come build their nests in this tall tree who was filled with joy and gratitude and her first squirrel friend became her ambassador and envoy to let all the other trees know that his tall free is not just the tallest but also the most amazing and awesome tree of the Wisconsin woods. And so, for so many years that came and gone, the tallest tree of the woods became the only tree where all the squirrels and birds that lived in these woods built their nests and stored their Winter food.

From then on the tallest tree, the squirrels, the birds and their babies lived happily forever in the woods of Wisconsin.

The Summer Camp Delight

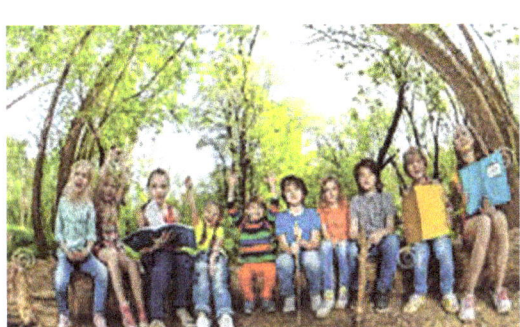

Atticus along with the other children who were in that Summer camp asked their coaches to repeat that story every night at their bedtime until they fell asleep. Their sleep was restful and uninterrupted. By the end of the 7th day of camping all the children had memorized that story.

When the children returned home from their Summer camp, they told the same story to their parents.

Since that special Summer camp, at bedtime every night, Atticus parents, told him the story of *The tallest tree in the woods of Wisconsin.* Constantly and expectedly, he would fall asleep and remained asleep until the next morning. He felt refreshed, happy and did not express feelings of sadness, or irritability. His aggressive and self -injurious behaviors seized and he ultimately excelled in his school achievements.

Teaching Diploma

It has been now 20 years, since Atticus participated in that Summer camp. He succeeded, and graduated from high school with honors, went to college and obtained a teaching diploma in special education. One of his successful teaching approach is based on the use of storytelling as a tool to communicate with children with *Autism Spectrum Disorder.*

Despite the passage of time and for many years past and present *The tallest tree in the woods of Wisconsin* remains one of Atticus favorite story to tell to all the children that he taught.

The End

* Segments previously published in; Khouzam HR. Storytelling Effects on Sleep Difficulties in Children with Autism Spectrum Disorders: Case Study. EC Neurology 11 (12), 2019.

TALE II

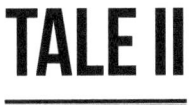

Kleptomania*

Oskar Schindler

Wounded soldiers returning from fighting in the jungles of Vietnam could die due to dwindling medical supplies. Bernise an Army nurse desperately needed bandages, tourniquets and surgical needles to mend and stitches the open wounds of injured soldiers. Her base had been depleted from these necessary devices. In another Army base there was an abundance of these medical supplies. In her younger years her father left her mother and her 2 younger sisters and never returned home. Her father succumbed to the perils and devastating effects of alcohol addiction. Her mother did her best to provide for her three daughters. Bernise remembered going to bed with unrelentless hunger pain. When she heard her sisters cry out from hunger pain, she would sneak out to a neighboring farmers market and skillfully steal fresh fruits and vegetables to share with her sisters. She was never caught and developed sophisticated techniques to even steal cooked meals that were sometimes served to the crowds who have frequented the farmers market.

Raiding the Bases

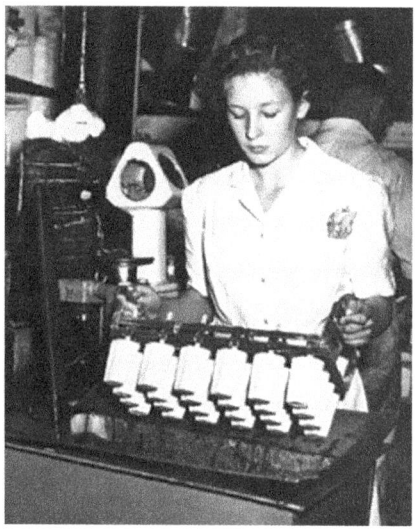

Bernise attempted and exhausted every possible means to solve the problem to no avail. She decided to visit other bases under the pretenses of cheering and encouraging the medics and nurses who were caring for the wounded. She then will carefully sneak to the storage areas and steal their surplus of medical supplies. Her undiscovered and successful stealing seemed to have ignited her childhood memories of stealing food to nurture her young sisters. She began to experience feelings of joy and elation with her stealing successes. Bernise felt helpless toward her stealing compulsions, which persisted after she returned from Vietnam. She was clinically diagnosed with kleptomania, and did not adhere with various therapeutic interventions which were provided by psychologists, and the attendance, of self-help groups, and counseling sessions.

Throwing the Spoil

Bernise never married and for 22 years has been living alone. She continued to steal and shoplift for many years without being caught. Each episode of stealing was usually associated with a brief spark of elation followed by unbearable and overwhelming feelings of guilt and disgust. She always got rid of the stolen objects by throwing them in public garbage dumpsters. One day she stole several bottles of baby food and because she did not have any need for them, she worried about getting caught, so she sneaked them into the shopping cart of another shopper who had already gone through the check out lane.

Who is Oscar Schindler?

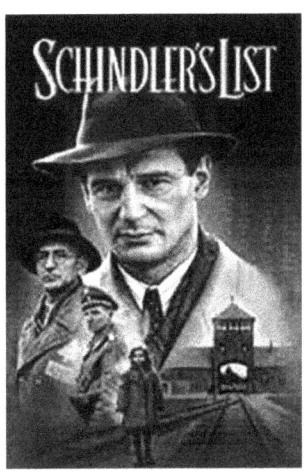

Subsequently that shopper was arrested by the police despite her innocence. Bernise felt guilty, terrified, and immobilized. She took a taxi cab to her apartment and thought of committing suicide by ingesting rat poison. As she was getting ready to mix the rat poison with her food she was distracted by a musical piece which was a prelude for a movie that was about to begin on her television screen. The movie was Schindler's List, which aroused her curiosity, and she temporarily abandoned her suicidal plan in order to watch it. Schindler's List, which was directed by Steven Spielberg is a 1994 Oscar-winning film that portrays Oskar Schindler, a German entrepreneur, who during the Holocaust had an unbeatable zeal for using Jewish individuals as cheap labor to maximize his profits. Being stricken by the sufferings of his workers, Schindler greed is transformed to compassion. The film had scenes of the Nazis stealing the possessions that were owned by the Jews. Some scenes portrayed the stealing of golden and silver teeth from the victims who were tortured and eventually murdered. Bernise identified with these Nazi thieves and felt overwhelmed with grief, guilt, and shame. She then realized that her acts of theft were a violation of God Eight's Commandment "Thou shall not steal". Rather than pursuing her suicide plan, she called a distant cousin who lived in another state and who happened to be a Christian pastor. She confessed to him and told him all her past history of shoplifting and stealing. He advised her to immediately return to the store to clear the innocent shopper and to surrender herself to the legal authorities.

Felony Charges and Redemption

The store had series of video recordings showing Bernise multiple previous stealing events. She was arrested, charged, tried and was sentenced to serve a jail term. During her incarceration she intensively studied the Bible. After completion of her sentence she enrolled in a Bible College and became an ordained assistant pastor. She was finally liberated from the affliction of kleptomania. She joined a group of prison ministers. She volunteered her time to visit women inmates who are serving jail sentences for various crimes. Bernise created a short Podcast presentation in which she narrates her own life experiences as examples to illustrate the role that her religious beliefs played in her redemption. She also sent letter to her former psychologist, psychiatrist and counselors in which she confirmed that she firmly believes that by internalizing her Christian faith she was relieved from kleptomania and from any suicidal contemplation. She also recommended to all her friends and acquaintances to have Schindler's List as must see movie!

* Segments previously published in; Khouzam HR, Williams L, Manzano N. Religion and Motion Pictures' Effects on Reversing Suicidal Intentions: Two Case Studies. *Psychological Reports*, 92:251-257, 2003.

TALE III

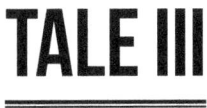

*Hidden Power**

Be mindful of what you say

S andra is a 68-year-old single, never married flower shop owner who had received several public recognitions for her outstanding special occasions flower arrangements. Unbeknown to her customers, she was always melancholic and had episodes of depression that required inpatient hospitalizations. During her last hospitalization, she walked into my office, closed the door, and uncontrollably wept. This was an unusual occurrence, since despite her pervasive melancholia, she always reflected an image of tenacity and stoicism. She was never heard or witnessed crying.

Tearfulness

Sensing my alarmed stare, Sandra sought to assure me and said that although medications "help a little, " pills cannot restore her lost self-esteem or reverse her constant feelings of impending doom. She then went on to say that her tears are not an expression of a deep feeling of sadness, but rather a manifestation of joy. She felt better now than when she was admitted to the hospital 3 weeks earlier, and that she was ready to return back to her home. As I echoed the word "ready", Sandra started to weep and apologized for losing control.

Negative Connotation

Among the clinical staff of the inpatient unit, there was a common perception about Sandra's character. She was known to detest the patients who weep. She insisted that tears are for the "needy" and "weak" especially when expressed in public. This dramatic change in Sandra's emotional display was worrisome. It could indicate an unreadiness for a hospital discharge. I asked Sandra if her tearfulness was provoked by the word "ready"! In response she sat back in her chair, crossed her arms, took a deep breath and loudly uttered "yes, yes, of course, isn't it obvious!"

Background Account

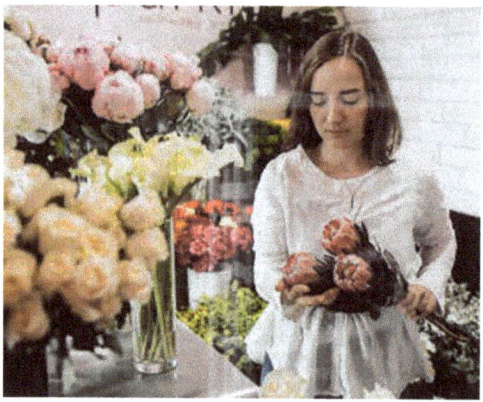

For the past 45 years Sandra felt invisible with no one noticing or acknowledging her existence. Although most of her customers admired and applauded her unique style of flower arrangements, she never received any personal compliment. The word that she repeatedly and constantly heard was, are the flowers "ready" to be picked up. All the tributes were bestowed on the flowers and never conveyed to her.

Enriched Vocabulary

I thought about alternative expression of readiness. I asked Sandra a hypothetical question. What would have happened if the customers used words such as "beautiful job" or "splendid" or "superb". With a big smile, She answered "Superb", that would be lovely. So I said, because of your "superb" participation in your treatment plan you will be able to return home. Her face brightened, she stood up straight, and said in an assertive and determined tone of voice "yes for sure, I am ready to leave the hospital and to return back home."

Pearl of Wisdom

Since that encounter with Sandra, along with colleagues, we embraced the inclusion and the use of words that are culturally associated with meaningful personal impact.

The notion that language contains information other than the speaker's immediate meaning should not be surprising to psychiatrists. One of the premises of psychiatry is that patients have important themes and concerns underlying what they say or hear. I remain forever grateful to Sandra who taught me a valuable lesson in rediscovering the hidden power of any spoken word.

* Segments previously published in; Khouzam HR. The Hidden Power of Words. Clinical Anecdote. *Clinical Psychiatry News* 20 (7): 17, 1992.

TALE IV

Unexpected Reunion

The Battle of the Bulge
&
The Battle of Anzio

The Battle of the Bulge, was the last major German offensive campaign on the Western Front during World War II. The battle lasted for five weeks from December 16, 1944 to January 1945. It was launched through the densely forested Ardennes region between Belgium and Luxembourg. The United States and British forces suffered from 77, 000 to more than 83, 000 losses, including at least 8, 600 fatal causalities. The "Bulge" was considered the largest and bloodiest single battle fought by the United States in World War II and is described as the third-deadliest campaign in American history.

The Battle of Anzio was a battle of the Italian Campaign of World War II that took place from January 22, 1944 to June 5, 1944 and ending with the capture of Rome. Although the operation was considered a success against the strong German Forces, the lives of so many soldiers were lost to achieve this crucial phase of the capture of Rome, Mussolini's strong hold.

Prisoner of War

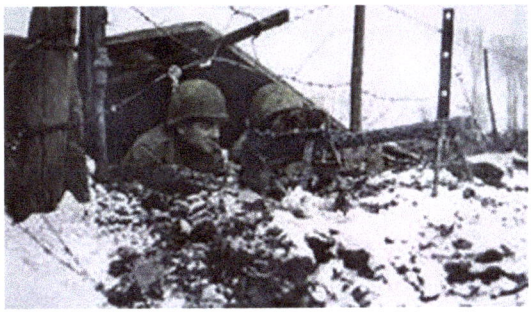

Jeremiah, a 92 year old World War II Veteran, fought during the Battle of the Bulge and taken as a Prisoner of War (POW). During his POW captivity, he was only allowed a small ration of water a day. He constantly felt thirsty and on several occasions fainted from the extreme thirst. His German guards thought that he was faking the fainting and subsequently further decreased his daily ration of water. When he returned back to the States, he married his neighbor, they have been close friend since grade school but the marriage lasted for 9 months and ended with a divorce. Although Jeremiah dearly loved his wife, she felt that he was cold, detached and unable to express his love and affection.

No Rest for the Weary

Jeremiah had difficulty falling asleep and staying asleep due to disturbing dreams and nightmares. He would frequently wake up in the middle of the night, thirsty and despite drinking excessive amounts of water, his thirst would not abate. His ability to focus, concentrate and to recall recent events significantly diminished, due to constant preoccupation with his POW experiences. He subsequently was incapable of maintaining any steady employment. He spent his inheritance with purchasing a trailer home, and moved to an isolated and remote mountainous area. He cut all personal communication with his siblings, and avoided all social activities. He drank excessively, using alcohol as a means to cope with his sleepless nights, the nightmares, and to quinch his constant thirst.

Overdose Attempt

On an anniversary date of his POW day of capture, he was overwhelmed with despair, hopelessness and had a pervasive sense of a foreshortened future. He decided that this was the day to end his earthly existence. He drank hard liquor all day, wishing to die from an alcohol overdose. He was found unconscious by an electric company electrician, who was conducting an annual maintenance check up in the region. He was admitted to an Intensive Care Unit (ICU) for observation and treatment. After 5 days of ICU care, he regained his consciousness. He was referred for a psychiatric evaluation and was assessed and diagnosed with posttraumatic stress disorder (PTSD). Fortunately he was able to achieve sobriety by his regular attendance of an Alcohol Anonymous(AA) group. He also joined a specialized PTSD care ttreatment (PCT) program.

Relentless Sleepless Nights

The AA attendance and the specialized PCT treatment had a positive effects on decreasing Jeremiah's social isolation and preventing alcohol use. His sleepless nights due to thirst, bad dreams and nightmares persisted. He was discouraged and stopped attending AA meeting and the PCT program. He felt hopeless and detached. His AA sponsor immediately contacted him and introduced him to Benjamin another World War II Veteran who fought during the Battle of Anzio in Italy. Benjamin invited Jeremiah to join a group of friends who were of similar age. The group met once a week at a nearby pancake and breakfast house. The group also traveled to national parks. Jeremiah was initially reluctant to participate in this group activities. Benjamin insistence and encouragement persuaded Jeremiah to visit the grand canyon.

Grand Canyon Surprise

Unexpectedly there was another group of veterans from a different state visiting the Grand Canyon. Jeremiah noticed a name tag of a veteran that was written in cursive. This attracted his attention and he drew near to read it. The name was Martin. For few seconds, he felt as if he was in a daze. He cleaned his eye glasses to assure that he read the name correctly. Could that be Martin his army buddy during the Battle of the Bulge. Yes, he was. They both thought that one of them died during that terrible merciless fight. It seemed that their union was heavenly ordained. Needless to say they spent the whole day reminiscing and relieving the countless memories they had since their boot camp training days. They exchanged addresses and promised to communicate on a regular basis and they kept that promise.

Friendship Rekindled

Over the following 3 months, Jeremiah and Martin rekindled their friendship and were communicating almost daily. Jeremiah noticed that he was able to sleep through the night. He was not disturbed by any bad dreams or nightmares. He found the weekly breakfast meeting with Benjamin and his group of veterans to be helpful in minimizing his social isolation and in providing an avenue for interacting and exchanging thoughts and ideas. He conveyed to Martin that meeting him has opened his closed mind and has enriched his soul with thankfulness and gratitude. He was finally able to enjoy restful nights, sweet dreams and freedom from thirst.

The National WWII Museum

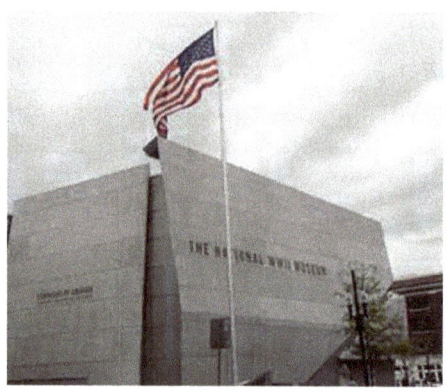

The National WWII Museum, formerly known as the National D-Day Museum, is a military history museum located in New Orleans, Louisiana, The museum focuses on the contribution made by the United States to Allied victory in World War II. Founded in 2000, it was later designated by the U. S. Congress as America's official National WWII Museum in 2004. The museum is a Smithsonian Institution affiliated museum, as part of the Smithsonian Institution's outreach program. The mission statement of the museum emphasizes the American experience in World War II. Martin's son in-law was one of the curator of the museum and asked him if he could share the harrowing accounts of the Battle of The Bulge to be displayed on one of the WWII pavilions.

Exhibit of Sacrifice and Valor

With decisiveness, confidence, and conviction, Jeremiah and Martin decided to relocate to New Orleans. Jeremiah sought a local volunteer organization assistance to refurbish his trailer home and it was mounted on wheels. Martin attached Jeremiah's trailer to his truck trailer home and together they traveled and eventually settled Jeremiah home in a New Orleans trailer Park. Over a period of 9 months they determinedly worked on designing and then constructing the special Battle of the Bulge exhibit in the National WWII museum. Impressed by their outstanding exhibit of Valor which attracted the attention and admiration of so many visitors. One of the museum inspector could not believe that this amazing artful and inspiring exhibit was designed and completed by two individuals who were in their golden years and in their nineties!!

Extending the invitation

The museum inspector thought that Jeremiah and Martin were retired architects or constructors. He was surprised when they clarified that they had no background or formal education in these domains. They then asked if he would like to have an exhibit about the Battle of Anzio. He unequivocally welcomed that proposal. They instantly reached Benjamin, who was delighted with such a prospect. He travelled to New Orleans where he resided with one of his distant cousin's home. Jeremiah, Martin, and Benjamin rolled their sleeve and over a course of 5 months designed and constructed a breath taking display of the Battle of Anzio at the National WWII Museum.

Living the Honorable Life

Jeremiah, Martin and Benjamin permanently resettled in New Orlenas. They volunteered to work at the National WWII Museum. They were a valuable asset and an unmatched source of historical facts about the crucial importance of the Battle of The Bulge and the Battle of Anzio. They escorted thousands of visitors and dignitaries to the exhibits and pavilions of the National WWII Museum in New Orleans. Although they are now in their mid-nineties, they are as vibrant as men in their twenties. They are now nicknamed the three valiant WW II heroes "*One for all and all for one*".

TALE V

Castleman Disease

The Sioux Tribe Timeless Wisdom

He could not bear it, as a medic, Conrad was unable to save his friend Calvin life during *the Battle for Fallujah* in Iraq. He wished he was the one who died and that Calvin would have lived and safely returned to his hometown in South Dakota. How would he face Calvin's parents, his sister, his wife and his 2 young sons. Conrad did not have a family, his parents had passed, he was the only child and never married. He had one paternal cousin Ewing who lived in Spain. Their relations has been strained since their late childhood years, when a conflict arose following his intentional dismantling of a personally designed remote controlled toy military tank.

The Joys of Childhood

As a little boy, Conrad was always cheerful and encouraging. His dad taught him how to design and create his own toys from discarded pieces of woods and metals. As his dad's apprentice he mastered the skills and art of welding. They made wooden remote controlled cartwheel, metal airplanes and toy trucks. Some were sold in local shops and county fairs. His parents loved their one and only child and he felt nurtured and joyfully fulfilled. His peaceful and enriched existence came to an unexpected crashing halt when his dad fell ill.

A Mysterious Illness

The doctors were baffled and they could not identify the cause of Conrad's father illness. It was accompanied by an elevated temperature which they labelled as fever of unknown origin or FUO. Despite elaborate and expensive investigations which exhausted all of his dad's savings, the FUO persisted to the dismay of all his treating physicians. Conrad's mom relentlessly spent countless sleepless nights surfing the world wide web looking for all possible causes of FUO. The day of an anticipated hospital discharge to a hospice care facility coincided with his dad's 45th birthday and his parents wedding anniversary. In the midst of his bewilderment, Conrad saw beams of fragmented light travelling across his bedroom window and pointing to the garage which was used as a storage area. He rushed and franticly pulled open the doors to search aimlessly the many stored and stocked books that were discarded from public libraries and purchased by his father who was an avid reader. A very old and dusty medical textbook with several torn and discolored pages seems to have been strangely shaken and fallen to the ground. He felt an inner sense of warmth and tranquility. The same feelings he had while sitting next to his grandpa who told him stories about the myths and stories of their Sioux tribe ancestors. His memory flashed back to his grandpa reminding him that kinship ties extend beyond human interaction and includes the natural and supernatural worlds. These two worlds are intimately related and represent a spiritual belief of how human beings should ideally act and relate to other humans, the natural world, the spiritual world, and to the cosmos and their impact on healing the soul, the mind and the body. So the cause of his dad's unexplained fever may lie within the pages of this old medical textbook. Feverishly he turned the dusty pages, which provoked uncontrollable sneezes and coughs. He feared that he may succumb to an asthma attack. He stopped turning the pages to catch his breath and realized that his eyes were mesmerized and fixated on an unfamiliar term *Castleman disease*, an illness that involves enlarged lymph nodes and fever. Could this disease be the cause of his dad's FUO. Jumping on his bike, and singing the superman theme lyrics" "faster than a speeding bullet! More powerful than a locomotive! Able to leap tall buildings at a single bound!". He arrived to the hospital while holding the old medical textbook and did not even greet his mom. He did not notice that she was sobbing. Two doctors dressed in long white coats were standing by his dad's beside. He showed them and shouted my dad's FUO is caused by *Castleman disease*. They seemed stunned, and the older grayed hair doctor uttered, it may be so my dear…it is too late. . your dad is gone!!!Grief stricken and flooded by an unbearable heart ache, he run to embrace his mom. Overwhelming sadness expressed in a river of tears never ended until she too departed from this world 3 months later on her 45th Birthday!

Semper Fi-Always Faithful-

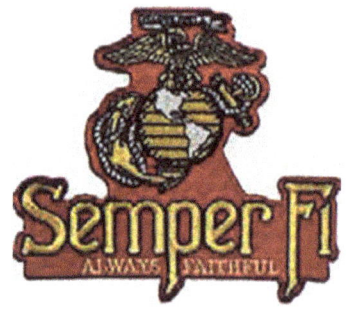

Devasted, despondent and in utter despair, Conrad was surrounded and cared for by his loving neighbors who considered him as the son that they never had. He was encouraged and nurtured and gradually regained his cheerful and joyful disposition and applied himself to study hard and became a paramedic, a vocation he chose to save those who are at risk of accidentally losing their life. He then joined the U. S. Marine Corps. He developed a strong bond and friendship with his newly found brotherhood of *Semper Fi* "Always faithful" Marines.

Thus began a new chapter of Conrad life as a medic and he did indeed save the life of so many wounded soldiers and civilians in Afghanistan and Iraq. He and Calvin were like brothers and always delighted in announcing that they are brothers from different mothers. Although they have never met prior to joining the Marines, they both grew up in two nearby towns in South Dakota. They also were able to trace their ancestry to the Sioux tribe. So after all they may be distant relatives. They were planning on exploring their lineage to find out if they have blood and genetic ties. In the brutal *Battle for Fallujah* many Marines suffered and died despite Conrad and other medics heroic endeavors to save the life of the fallen soldiers. Calvin died from profuse bleeding that defied all of Conrad unmatched skills and tireless efforts to stop the bleeding. His tour in Iraq is approaching its completion and he will be returning back to his home town in South Dakota where Calvin's family resides.

Meeting with the Loved Ones

Long sleepless nights reemerged and triggered the painful memories of losing his dad possibly to **Castleman Disease** and his mom to her overwhelming grief. He remembered his grandpa whispering that the Sioux do not have a fear of death or of going to an underworld. They do believe in a spirit world (Wakan Tanka) in the sky in which the deceased are free of pain and suffering. This remembrance ignited a sense of power and resolve and he felt an inner calling to reach out to Calvin's family and he did. He was surprised by their serene and welcoming attitude. He was embraced by Calvin's parents and his sister, although they have never met, they seem to have intimately known him. They encouraged him and accompanied him to meet Calvin's widow and his 2 sons. The youngest son, Calvin Junior was uncontrollably screaming and throwing a tantrum temper. Earlier that day his older brother had accidentally broke his remote controlled drone which he has received as Christmas gift from his father. Consolation poured out from everyone, but Calvin Junior relentlessly maintained his steady stream of screaming. A Sioux tribe pearl of wisdom unexpectedly jumped into Conrad's conscious awareness. He clearly recalled hearing an adage "rediscover the soul-stirring forces all around you". His mind flashed back to his childhood years and to the exact event when he intentionally dismantled his cousin's

Ewing personally designed remote controlled toy tank. Could this be a soul-stirring memory that is provoking him to contact Ewing. Without hesitation he told Calvin Junior that he has a cousin who lives in Spain and he could repair the drone. He needed few days to search for his contact information. Silence and quietness engulfed everyone presence. The screaming abruptly stopped.

Finding the Estranged Cousin

Three long days of tireless efforts in searching the internet and social media outlets yielded Ewing's address in Spain. Torn between hesitation and determination, Conrad contacted Ewing who was in hospital bed recovering from a successful treatment of *Castleman disease!!*. Was this a mere coincidence or a providential soul-stirring phenomenon?? Sharing about his dad succumbing to that awful illness and Ewing healing mended years of heartaches and separation. Ewing then revealed that he wished he could have died from that illness, because after 3 years of dating, his fiancée called off their planned wedding without any reasonable explanation. Conrad felt his cousin sadness and despair, these familiar emotions that had accompanied his life since he lost his parents which were then magnified with Calvin's death. He offered Ewing an open invitation to visit him in South Dakota their Sioux tribe ancestral land. Ewing also drew with meticulous details, the many steps that would be needed to repair Calvin's junior remote controlled drone and send them via his smart phone as a screen shot.

How Could It Be!

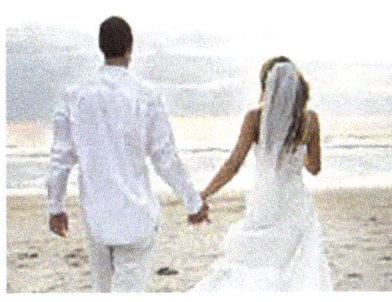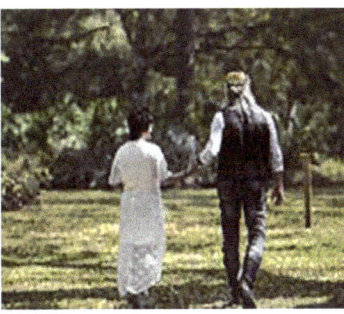

Three months later and without any advance notice, Ewing was knocking on Conrad front door. What ensued could be described as a magical fairy tale except for the fact that it really happened. Calvin's widow and her two sons instantly fell in love with Ewing. Calvin sister who never married or dated because she wanted to devote her life to the care of her elderly parents did fall in love with Conrad. Double weddings were performed and blessed on the same date that coincided with the date of Conrad's parents wedding. Calvin's widow, Henrietta now Ewing's wife set foot along with her two sons on a boarding flight to Spain their new homeland destination. Conrad with his bride Calvin's sister, Anatolia purchased a land in South Dakota and began building a house that will be large enough to accommodate them along with Calvin and Anatolia parents.

Despite the tragic and untimely deaths inflicted by *Castleman disease* in South Dakota and the *Battle for Fallujah* in Iraq; the Sioux tribe timeless wisdom was the guiding path that converted lives which were shattered by grief and despair to renewed and enduring wonderful lives.

TALE VI

*Shared Delusional Disorder**
The Age of the COVID -19 Pandemic

Everett a 41-years-old construction worker, was admitted to the hospital due to fever with chills, cough, difficulty breathing, fatigue with muscle aches, headache, sore throat and runny nose. He tested positive for a COVID-19 infection. He was discharged from the hospital after receiving 9 days of medical support and oxygen therapy. A week later, Everett's wife reported that he was behaving very strangely. He became delusional and suspicious. He firmly believed that his neighbors were plotting to kill him and his family using the nerve gas, sarin, which he felt was supplied by terrorists. He began to implement extreme precautionary actions by barricading himself in their apartment and barb wired his front door entrance. He also ordered various chemicals from online dark websites with the intention of using them as antidotes to the nerve gas, sarin.

Unusual Behaviors

As a result of these sudden behavioral changes, his wife begged him to visit his primary care physician. He had a complete physical examination which did not reveal any abnormal findings. He had no symptoms or signs of COVID-19 reinfection, inflammation, head injury, bone fractures or joint problems. His lab tests, , were all normal. Due to his healthy physical condition, no further medical work up or imaging study was recommended. He was not offered any treatment. His wife and his two12-years-old twin daughters all fortunately tested negative for COVID-19 infection. His wife sought help and support from several of his family members and friends. They were residing out of state and unable to come to help and persuade him to abandon his strange behavior and bizarre delusions.

Everett had a very close friend, Fabian, whom he had known since they were on the baseball team in high school. Everett and Fabian shared a very strong friendship, and many of their classmates had mistakenly thought that they were biological brothers. They have kept close contact throughout the years, and they were each other "best men" in their respective weddings. Their families travelled together and camped in national parks every summer and special anniversary dates. Due to COVID-19 pandemic restrictions and social distancing precautions, the two families have not gathered for a long time and only kept in touch via social media and face time. Everett's wife reached out to Fabian and pleaded with him to intervene and persuade his lifelong friend to "gain back his sanity." Fabian agreed to help but he first wanted to carefully analyze and investigate the "whole situation" before he could intervene.

A Miraculous Change

Everett had no knowledge of his wife's arrangement with Fabian. Suddenly and for no known reason, Everett expressed a dramatic change in his behaviour. He apologized for his unusual actions and reported that all his fears and suspiciousness were kind of "a bad dream." He continued to improve over the course of the following three weeks, and he regained his normal level of physical and psychological functioning.

In the meantime, Fabian 's wife contacted Everett to inform him that her husband has lost his mind and was acting strangely over the past three weeks. She described him as being suspicious and fearful. He exhibited bizarre belief about a terrorist plot planned by their neighbors to spread the nerve gas sarin in their place of residence. He barricaded himself and barb wired their front door entrance. He also checked the online dark websites for chemicals and antidotes to the nerve gas sarin! Everett was alarmed and became extremely concerned about Fabian's wellbeing and tried to convince him that he is just having the exact same "bad dream" that himself has gone through due his contracting the COVID-19 infection. In response, Fabian became very angry, hostile and threatened to retaliate and to harm Everett and his whole family.

A Friend's Description

Fabian owned a hardware store. He was a fit and healthy gentleman. He did not smoke or used any caffeine, alcohol, illicit or recreational drugs. He tested negative for COVID-19 but was deemed a potential danger for self and others. As result of his threatening behavior toward Everett's family, he was involuntarily hospitalized in a psychiatric emergency unit and was treated with an antipsychotic medication. He responded well to that treatment. His bizarre belief about a terrorist plot that was planned by the neighbors to spread the nerve gas sarin in his place of residence subsided, He regained his insight and could not believe that he acted and behaved in such bizarre manners. He was then discharged from the psychiatric unit and returned back to his home. Fabian then reached out and apologized to Everett and his family, and they rekindled their enduring and cherished friendship.

Explaining the Puzzle

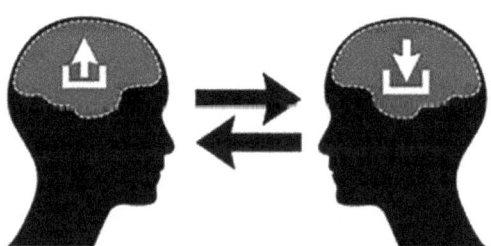

The condition that Fabian developed is called shared delusional disorder (SDD). While SDD is considered a rare psychiatric disorder, it was historically described as Folie à deux ('madness for two'), also known as shared psychosis or induced delusional disorder. When it affects more than two people, it may be called folie à. . . trois ('three') or quatre ('four'); and further, folie en famille ('family madness') or even folie à plusieurs ('madness of several'). The disorder was first conceptualized in France in the 19th century by Charles Lasègue and Jean-Pierre Falret, hence also known as Lasègue-Falret syndrome. This disorder is most commonly diagnosed when two or more individuals live in proximity, may be socially or physically isolated, and have little interaction with other people. SDD is characterized by symptoms of delusional beliefs, and sometimes hallucinations that are transmitted from one individual to another. The treatment of SDD usually require the isolation of the individuals who share the same delusions and monitoring if the delusion resolves or lessens over time. This intervention was not necessary since Everett and Fabian were already geographically separated from each other. Everett did not require treatment with an antipsychotic medication since his delusions were spontaneously resolved following his recovery from the COVID-19 infection. Conversely Fabian who did not contract COVID-19, had a persistence of symptoms as a result of developing SSD thus requiring treatment with an antipsychotic medication.

COVID-19 Impact on Mental Stability

It seemed that Everett developed his first episode of psychotic symptoms manifested by delusions as a complication of COVID-19 infection which was also associated with social isolation and decreased human interactions imposed by the pandemic guidelines. While these measures are necessary to prevent infections spread and are lifesaving, living in quarantine and socially distancing oneself has been known to trigger psychotic episodes, particularly in vulnerable individuals. Both Everett and Fabian, were emotionally and psychologically stable individuals prior to the COVID-19 pandemic; they did not have any family history of psychiatric or emotional conditions; and at the time, they were not living in close proximity. So, it is still unclear if their psychotic symptoms were direct consequence of COVID-19 pandemic impact on their mental stability.

Good News

The treatment with an antipsychotic medication was clinically indicated and urgently warranted to prevent Fabian from developing more complications that are associated with an untreated SDD. That treatment was successful and led to the remission of the delusion without the development of any adverse effect. Although it remains unclear if the SDD would have resolved spontaneously with the passage of time. Clinical data about the prognosis of rare conditions such as SSD, are currently lacking, and it is expected that the majority of cases go unreported. However, in Fabian's case, the treatment with an antipsychotic medication seemed to have achieved a desirable effect and contributed to the recovery from his SDD.

* Segments previously published in; Khouzam HR, Tran J. Cariprazine Treatment of Shared Delusional Disorder in the Age COVID -19: A Case Report. *Journal of Clinical Cases & Reports.* (S12):7 -13, 2022.

TALE VII

Existential Depression *

A Father and Son Unbreakable Bond

Dennis, a Korean War veteran, recalled that when he was seven years old he played with wooden toy soldiers and dreamed that one day he would be a real soldier, and would fight in real battles to defend his country. Although he had difficulties with reading and writing, and was considered illiterate, he volunteered and joined the US Army. His heroic achievements during the Korean War earned him several medals of honor. He was suffering from posttraumatic stress disorder (PTSD) which at the time of the Korean war (was called Combat Fatigue or Soldier's Heart). He had recurrent intensive recollections of combat experiences, distressing frightening dreams in addition to persistent feelings of detachment and estrangement that led to two failed marriages. He has been married to his third wife for eleven years and had a ten year old son whom he named Teddy.

Son Love For His Daddy

Dennis recalled that when Teddy was four years old, he wanted his daddy to read to him bedtime stories. Due to his illiteracy, such a request irritated him, made him angry, and he became severely depressed. Teddy subsequently changed his requests to watching home videos instead of reading. In the video "The Little Engine That Could" a little train, with a heavy cargo of animals, while trying to climb a snowy mountain, kept repeating the phrase, "I think I can, I think I can, " and eventually managed to reach its destination. Teddy commented that if the little engine could climb the mountain, then his daddy could learn to read. Touched by his son's endearment, Dennis then enrolled in an adult school, earned a high school diploma, and felt connected to his nuclear family, while still experiencing detachment and estrangement from others.

Pinocchio and His Courage

When Teddy was seven years old he enjoyed engaging his daddy in playing with wooden toy soldiers. However, such interactive play triggered Dennis PTSD symptoms and he relapsed into a long period of severe depression. Teddy stopped playing with the toy soldiers and instead watched a video of the animation picture "Pinocchio" with his father. In that movie Pinocchio was magically changed from a wooden toy into a real living boy after he proved himself to be honest and courageous like his daddy. Subsequent to these comments, the PTSD symptoms of depression subsided. Dennis was encouraged and was filled with enthusiasm and enrolled in college in the hope of becoming a civil engineer. At the age of ten, Teddy was an outstanding soccer player. However, the noises, the crowd, and the excitement of soccer games triggered PTSD thus, preventing his father from attending most of Teddy's final games. Teddy's team was the winning team of the season, and he was given as a gift a video about Jesse Owens.

Jesse Owens

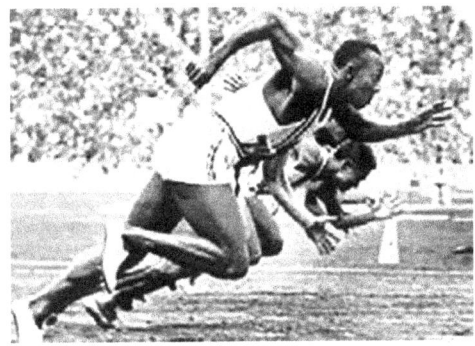

Teddy and his daddy sat together to watch Jesse Owens. The movie was a documentary about this phenomenal American track-and-field athlete who set a world record in the running broad jump (also called long jump) that stood the record for 25 years. Jesse Owens, also won four gold medals at the 1936 Olympic Games in Berlin, Germany. His four Olympic victories were a blow to Adolf Hitler's intention to use the Games to show off the superiority of the Aryan race. Teddy commented to his daddy that he reminded him of Jesse Owens. Inspired by the movie and Teddy's comments, Dennis decided to change his major courses of study from civil engineering to psychology.

Depression: An introduction

In a course assignment, Dennis wrote an essay about "Existential Depression" in which he described how PTSD led him to live in an existential vacuum; that was devoid from meanings. He was then stricken by feelings of helplessness and hopelessness. As he continued to ponder on the meaningless of his life, he increasingly realized that life itself was the cause of his depression, and thought that if life came to an end, then depression would end. He was baffled by the facts that some people escape such an existential depression, while others are completely engulfed by it. Dennis, then concluded that the causes of his depression were not causes at all but rather excuses to justify being depressed, and that his son's relentless engagement, and his selection of uplifting comments were essential in bringing meaning back to his life, and hence defeated his existential depression.

The Passage

Convinced by this newly found thoughts he began the process of reconnecting with his extended family. He reached out and asked forgiveness from the victims of his 2 previous failed marriages. He completed his courses of study in psychology and became a counselor that specialized in helping those who suffer from PTSD and existential depression. Teddy grew up and went to college and graduated with a degree in public communication. He became a narrator of many documentaries that especially focused on the plight of those who are afflicted with the aftermath of emotional trauma and depression. In his documentary debut, his daddy Dennis along with his behind the scene heroine, his mum Alice (the sunshine of their family) were his guests of honor.

* Segments previously published in; Khouzam HR. Existential Depression. The Newsletter of the New Hampshire Psychiatric Society *Psychiatric Viewpoint* Issue 1:5-6, Summer 1997.

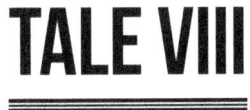

TALE VIII

*Misspelled Word**

Crisis Averted

After a long day of working at the crisis intervention center. I finally caught up with typed the electronic record clinical notes, checked any outstanding laboratory values, and completed the arduous task of completing multidisciplinary treatment plans. Now, at 4:30 p. m., just as the thought of reading some recent psychiatric literature passed through my mind, I was paged for a code purple—a psychiatric emergency.

Knock-Knock-Who is There?

Greg, a 29-year-old gentleman, was in the emergency room—handcuffed, attended by a police officer, and accompanied by his wife, two older brothers, and his grandmother. Earlier that day, Greg, had shot several newly planted trees in his neighbor's front yard with a BB gun. The neighbor and all of Greg's family members had failed to persuade him to stop this irrational behavior. The police were called, and Greg was handcuffed and brought to the emergency room. According to the family, there was no precedent for such an action, and he had no history of psychiatric or substance use conditions. His family history was also negative for psychiatric disorders.

Eerie Appearance

Greg was calm and appeared to be unconcerned about the day's events. He countered my attempts to interview him with absolute silence. He kept gesturing to the police officer that he wanted the handcuffs to be removed. I saw his request as a golden opportunity to show empathy. My request to fulfill his wishes was answered by a clear and loud "No" from the police officer, Greg's family, and the emergency room nursing staff. My mind went numb as I attempted to review any possible diagnosis of this condition. All I could think of was to rule out "not otherwise specified" diagnoses. His grandmother kept asking, "What are you going to do to my baby?" His wife was enraged by that statement and shouted, "he is not a baby; we are expecting our first baby soon!" His brothers joined the debate and confirmed that Greg had always been "Grandma's baby." I was at a loss on how to intervene, and the police officer, seeming to lose his patience, asked in a clear, firm, and raspy tone of voice, "What's your recommendation, Doc?"

Do Not Know What To Do

I was overwhelmed with anxiety. I then vividly remembered a therapeutic pearl of wisdom : "Be courteous and considerate, and intervene with several options without escalating anxiety and fears." So I came closer to Greg and in a soft voice asked, "Could you please tell me what you were doing with that wee wee gun?"

A burst of laughter engulfed everyone present, including Greg, who then became teary eyed. He graciously asked his wife to hold him. She hugged and kissed him. He then uttered, "Honey, I'm so glad you're going to be our baby's mom." The grandmother and the two brothers showered the couple with hugs and kisses. The police officer smoothly and quietly removed the handcuffs.

Unintended Error

Greg approached me and loudly announced that I "did pull a fast one" on him and that the words "wee wee gun" pulled him out of his confusion. Only then did I realize that because of my anxiety, I had said "wee wee" instead of "BB" gun. Greg's wife, his grandmother, and his two brothers tearfully thanked me for bringing him back to reality. The police officer and the emergency room nursing staff congratulated me for skillfully handling a potentially violent patient.

I wanted to clarify my mistake and explain that saying "wee wee" was not intentional. Then I recalled that in psychotherapy, affirmation is a simple intervention that involves supportive comments like yes, no, or uh-huh, so I said "uh-huh." Immediately Greg proceeded to tell me that when he was six years old, his father promised to buy him a BB gun when he reaches his 18th birthday. Unfortunately, his father lost his job a month before that birthday, and he never got the promised BB gun. Although he did not harbor any resentment toward his father, he felt disappointed and "betrayed." He also made a conscious determination that when he became a father, he would never promise his children any gifts unless he had already purchased them.

Purchase of a BB gun

When Greg found out a few days before the shooting incident that he and his wife were going to have a baby, he felt numb. He could not remember the reason that led to the purchase of the BB gun or the antecedents of his emergency room visit.

By then I felt calm and collected and thought that this was the opportunity to obtain a detailed history and a mental status examination, to help confirm a probable *case* of psychogenic amnesia. Neither Greg nor his family were interested in such an endeavor. They agreed to come for a follow-up appointment, they thanked me for my help, and they all left in a joyful mood. I was left alone with the police officer, who suddenly stood up, shook my hand, and said I was a "great psych doc." However, the emergency room nursing staff expressed their dismay at the ending of the intervention, as no medications had been prescribed.

Documentation Dilemma

I concluded Greg's clinical note with the statement that the source of his apparently irrational and otherwise inexplicable behavior seemed to be in a part of his mind of which he was not consciously aware. I then realized that Greg's behaviors and my reactions to them were expressions of interacting conscious and unconscious processes. My situational anxiety had led to the unconscious use of "wee wee," and that humorous term apparently evoked conscious and unconscious memories from Greg's childhood that were related to his expected fatherhood. At that moment my enthusiasm for dynamic psychiatry was rekindled.

I then also realized that considerable time had passed, and that according to mandated clinical guidelines for seeing patients, my clinical intervention would be categorized as "disproportionately costly." The introduction of practice guidelines that are focused on productivity, had pushed clinicians to squeeze more patients into increasingly shorter time slots. Under the banner of cost-effectiveness, psychiatrists are constantly urged, and at times pressured, to limit interactions with patients to the task of prescribing psychotropic medications and to refer them to other mental health professionals if they need psychotherapy.

Back To Dynamic Psychiatry

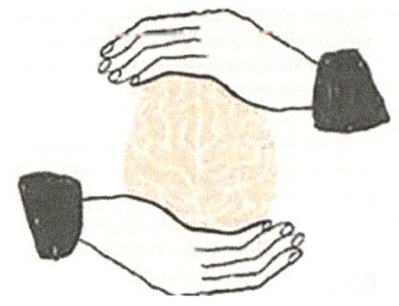

I returned back to my office and looked for my textbooks on dynamic psychiatry. They were at the bottom of a cardboard box that I had not opened for few years. They now stand clean, tall, and proud, on my bookshelves.

Although not formally expressed at the time I am forever thankful to Greg and his family. Their crisis situation galvanized me to take a conscious step to reintegrate dynamic psychiatry into the treatment of all the patients that I am privileged to evaluate and treat.

* Segments previously published in; Khouzam HR. A Touch of Dynamic Psychiatry. *Psychiatric Services* 51: 437-438, 2000.

TALE IX

Dyslexia

A Broken Back

A majority of the 101st Airborne Division's tactical operations were performed in the Central Highlands and in the A Shau Valley during the Vietnam War. Among its major operations was the vicious battle to retake Ap Bia Mountain, also known as "Hamburger Hill" battle. During the Vietnam war, troopers from the 101st won 17 Medals of Honor for combat bravery. This courageous division according to many estimates lost almost 20, 000 soldiers who were either killed or wounded in action in Vietnam which is more than twice of the 9, 328 casualties that occurred in World War II. Harold survived "Hamburger Hill" battle at a great cost of braking his back.

Addicted to Pain Killers

He returned home with shattered dreams of running his family construction business.

He felt like an invalid and physically disable. Any slight movement would evoke back pain. Opiates also known as "pain killers" seemed to be unmatched in their effects on alleviating his back pain. Eventually Harold used excessive amount of these medications and exceeded the maximum amount that was allowed by his prescribing doctors. He became addicted to these medications and all of his daily activities evolved around acquiring these pain killers even if he has to purchase them illegally on the streets of New York City from law breakers drug dealers.

He abandoned his deeply rooted moral values and became a mule for drug dealers agreeing to transport illegal drugs on behalf of the drug dealers as a mean to have an income to supplement his needs for the drugs.

Beaten to Death

Fed up with his life, he contemplated suicide by a drug overdose. Harold stole a large bag from his drug dealer and intended on injecting them with a needle while laying down in a street back alley which was one of the drugs addict hub in New York City. The drug dealer realized that a theft had occurred. Along with many street thugs they surrounded and severely beaten him with iron rods and baseball bats and left him for dead.

The Brooklyn VA Medical Center

Fortunately he had kept his Vietnam War Dog Tag which was identified by the police officers who were called by a passerby. Harold was brought to a local emergency room and with intensive care he was able to survive despite massive bleeding and a head concussion. During a rehabilitation drug addiction program assessment session, Harold was found to also have Dyslexia. This condition had made him reluctant to utilizing his GI educational benefits to enroll in school following his return from the Vietnam War. A speech and language pathology student who was completing her internship at that hospital where Harold was admitted for intensive care treatment felt drawn to assist him with his hospital discharge plans as he reminded her of her grandfather who was an Army Vietnam War Veteran and who was a volunteer at the same hospital. Her grandfather role was to use wheelchairs to transport patients between various hospital departments. The student Inez contacted her grandfather Jayden and asked if he could come and spend sometimes with Harold. Jayden introduced Harold to a myriad of services that are provided by the Veteran Hospital (also named VA Hospital) to veterans and upon his discharge from the recovery service he personally escorted him to the Brooklyn VA Medical Center.

Dyslexia in the Forefront

Despite many erected barriers and resistance to receive any help. Harold finally accepted to enter a VA Drugs rehabilitation treatment program. He received alternative pain management interventions that did not include opioids, he also received physical therapy to strengthen his back. He was enrolled in the homeless program which offered him the opportunity to get off the street and eventually acquired a permanent housing in a two bedrooms apartment in a near proximity to where his parents were still living. Although his parents were in their mid-eighties, his father was still operating the construction company that he owned. Inez the student pursued all the **preliminary** steps that were needed to refer Harold for dyslexia treatment at the Brooklyn VA Medical Center.

Individuals Who Overcame Dyslexia

One of the therapist suggested the attendance of group sessions that explored the life of historical characters and famous individuals with Dyslexia. He was surprised to know that several of his favorite and esteemed individuals such as Walt Disney, Pablo Picasso, Albert Einstein and Winston Churchill had dyslexia and they did overcome it by mastering and practicing their innate talents. Inspired by these findings, Harold decided to study drafting for construction of skyscrapers. Rather than bemoaning the fact that his broken back was a hindrance for construction. He relabeled his back as being his back bone instead of being a broken back.

Subsequently he became his dad's construction company CEO. He did not have to use his back to bend and stretch during construction projects. His back bone supported his body during his drafting and drawing of newly designed New York City skyscrapers.

Backbone Cherished

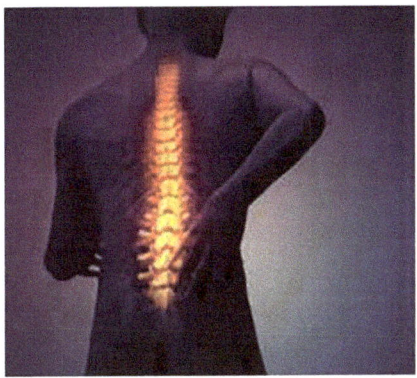

Total freedom from back pain was a far reaching desire. The pain would come and go and at times its occurrence was agonizing. He ingrained his soul with the mantra of cherishing his back despite the pain. On his father 90th birthday, Harold planned and executed a lavish party and invited many New York City dignitaries who were residing in some of the skyscrapers that his dad's company has contributed to their construction. He also invited Jayden, Inez and their families and many veterans that he met at the Brooklyn VA Medical Center, and who were afflicted with long lasting back pain. He designed special banners and dining table ornaments with beautiful inscriptions of his personal mantra. The mantra illustrated his faulty perception of his back as being a bad back. Conversely his back bone sustained his livelihood and allowed his innate talents to be expressed in drafting and drawing many of New York City breathtaking skyscrapers.

TALE X

*Practice Without a License**
No Good Deed Shall Escape Punishment

Following completion of my third year of medical school in Cairo, Egypt, I took a year off. During that year I worked odd jobs. While in London, I found a job as a waiter in a restaurant. One foggy evening in late spring, I was returning home to my apartment, still dressed in my waiter's uniform (a shiny, pink jacket with black lapels and cuffs). I noticed a frail, elderly lady walking her white, well-groomed poodle. For no apparent reason, the dog pulled the woman toward me. She followed, and the poodle jumped over and started sniffing my waiter's uniform.

Convulsive Seizure

While attempting to apologize for her dog's unexpected behavior, the lady began to hyperventilate. Her face turned blue, her whole body start shaking, and had a convulsive seizure. I took my jacket off and placed on the ground, gently held her head and slowly dropped her on the jacket to prevent her fall on the concrete pavement. My garment was used as ta pillow for her head. I made sure that her airways were opened and vigilantly monitored her pulse and respiratory rate. She lost consciousness and had a generalized seizure.

Foggy Evening

The poodle began licking me, drooling, and adding more fog to my eyeglasses. Unexpectedly, a young couple emerged from the fog. They noticed the situation and called for help. A few long minutes passed before a police car appeared on the scene. A constable emerged from the vehicle and introduced himself. Then, he proceeded to ask me if I robbed the woman and then knocked her down! I was at a loss for words. The woman stopped seizing and regained consciousness. She looked dazed and confused. Concerned about the poodle, she called out: "Laddie, laddie, my precious boy! Where are you?"

Just About to be Handcuffed

The constable was about to place me in handcuffs. The young couple proceeded to explain what they witnessed. The foggy weather was clearing up. Laddie appeared from nowhere and jumped into the lady's arms. She explained to the constable that she takes seizure medications and probably forgot to take her afternoon pill because Laddie wanted to go for the routine evening a walk!

Are you Licensed ?

The constable took the handcuffs away and asked me if I was a doctor. I told him that I was a medical student and he seemed pleased. He then asked me where I attended medical school. When he heard it was Cairo University, his face turned red. In a loud and authoritarian manner, he said, "In this country, you cannot practice medicine without a license." He then added, "This is your only and last chance before you get arrested for practicing without a license." He left the scene, grumbling all the way back to his police car.

The Effects of Fog

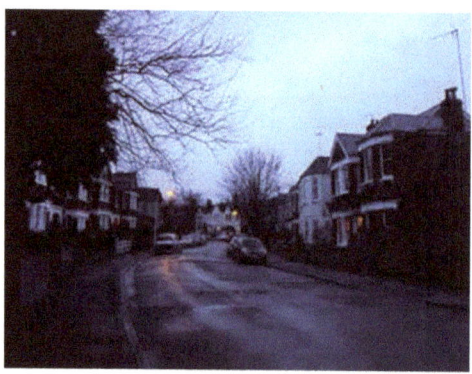

The Lady thanked me for my intervention, and Laddie fetched my jacket and dropped it at my feet. The young couple apologized for the constable's behavior. From then on, I never left the restaurant where I worked wearing my uniform. To this day, I get nervous every time I see fog, an elderly woman with a poodle, or a young couple holding hands.

Segments previously published in; Khouzam HR. Practice without a License, *Hospital Physician* 40(9):51, 2004.

TALE XI

*A Narrative of Giving**

The Children Will Survive - The Village Shall Prosper

His name was Ronnie. His parents called him Ronnie Runabout and nicknamed him "Run Ronnie Run." He was constantly reminded that he ran before he walked. At the age of 11 months, he was running everywhere, and no one could stop him to teach him how to walk.

Adopted at Birth

Ronnie was a lovely little boy who was adopted by a childless couple, after the tragic death of his parents in a house fire. He was told that his ancestors were Native Americans from New England. With immigrants settling to the New World, his ancestor's tribe, lost its identity and distinct culture. Ronnie adoptive parents were Anglo-Saxon Protestants with a sense of pride, honor and valor. They were established and settled in the foothills of the North-Eastern Mountains. They managed a ski resort in the Fall and Winter; and operated a quaint bed and breakfast during the Spring and Summer. Ronnie became the joy and the center of his parents' life. Due to his unmatched ability to run, his parents thought that he would become a famous athlete and one day competes in the Olympics as a track and field runner. Throughout his school years, Ronnie competed in many races and won them all. He had a dream that one day he would run and win the Olympic Marathon.

Tragedy Struck

At the age of 18, Ronnie's parents died in a car accident by a drunken driver, as the sole heir, he inherited all their wealth including the prime skiing hills, the bed and breakfast accommodation, and a twelve acres mansion. Ronnie, however was devastated by his parents' death. He stopped running and did not go to school for weeks. He was not eating and became extremely weak and emaciated. At that time, he had a high school friend named Denise. She was also a ballerina and was described as the prettiest girl in her class. She dearly loved and cherished Ronnie but never told him. She was quiet and reserved. She did not tell him that every night she dreamt of dancing with him. When Ronnie sank deep in his grief, Denise told her parents. They went with her to his mansion and told him how dearly and fondly Denise loved him. This love brought hope back to Ronnie's life. He resumed his schooling. Denise beautiful golden-reddish hair inspired Ronnie to call her the 'sunlight of his darkest days'. Ronnie graduated from high school with academic and athletic honors. He was offered scholarships to join prestigious Ivy League Universities.

Ronnie's parents had raised him as a generous giver. He declined the scholarships, and volunteered to join the Peace Corps. He was sent to work in the mountainous and unforgiving icy cold regions of Nepal. His exemplary and excellent performance gained him the highest degree of respect by his fellow volunteers and supervisors.

Winter in Nepal

On a Winter day with ice and frozen rain surrounding their wooden cabin, Ronnie and his closest friend almost froze to death when their cabin was swallowed by a raging avalanche. They were later rescued, they both had severe hypothermia. Ronnie suffered a frostbite that caused the amputation of all his toes. He was discharged from the Peace Corps with the highest recommendations and praises. Sadness and depression accompanied his journey home. He could no longer run. For Ronnie, running was living. He felt that without running his life lost its luster. In the midst of it all, Denise had remained his shining light of hope.

Unexpected News

He returned to his hilly estate, his mansion and his bed and breakfast. He realized that he had all this wealth awaiting him and contemplated the idea of beginning a new life journey without running. There was no one to welcome him home and even Denise wasn't there to welcome him home. Astonished, shocked and surprised, he wondered what could have happened. Hanging on his front porch there was a little note posted on his door. He opened it; and in it was a 'Dear John letter' from Denise. Before catching his breath, he limped as fast as he could to find what had happened. When he reached Denise home, other people that he did not know were living there. He was told that they recently bought that house and that Denise was engaged, to be married in a month to a friend that she met during Ronnie's service in Nepal.

Devastation

Ronnie became deeply sorrowful. He had come back to an empty home surrounded by twenty acres of beautiful hills, materially wealthy but friendless without a family. His sunlight Denise is gone forever. He lost hope and meaning and his life once again lost its luster. One day while contemplating suicide, he felt that his parents' spirit were whispering songs of hope, and urging him never to give up. He even heard "Ronnie Runabout Run Ronnie Run." He was seized by a divine love. He rediscovered the awe-inspiring beauty surrounding his home. A deer would walk by and look through the window of his kitchen. A wild turkcy would be attempting to fly over his roof. A bear brought newly born cubs and dropped them at Ronnie's feet. Ronnie gained a new meaning for his desperate life. He trusted nature with its majestic beauty and wild animals. He decided not to seek out people but to live a solitary life surrounded by his hills, woods and wild animals.

Doctor's Kindness

Ronnie lived seemingly content for several years until one morning he awakened with a sharp pain on the right side of his belly. The pain was so **excruciating**, that he couldn't breathe. He was transported by an ambulance to the nearby hospital. After a, thorough evaluation the examining doctor concluded that there was no serious medical reason for the pain and it resolved. Ronnie was deeply moved by the doctor's kindness. He noticed that the doctor had next to his name tag a lapel pin that read "God is Love". He felt a deep sense of calm and a new cause for reflection. He asked" How can I find God's love?" and after few moments of silence he humbly requested the doctor to pray for him. The doctor said I will pray for you so you can experience God love as described in His written words in the Bible. Ronnie then remembered that he had a Bible at home which he received as a gift from his parents when he was baptized during a youth camp. He felt a sense of joy and peace engulfing his being. He thanked the doctor and asked him to keep him in his prayers.

Never Take More Than What You Give

On his way home, Ronnie felt a sense of love engulfing all of his being. He realized that life is short, at 65 years of age he had been living a solitary and lonely life, which had been self-centered and self - preserving. As he read the Bible the words became alive" he who gains his life must lose it", "give", "serve", "tell" and "you are forgiven", "for by Christ's wounds you are healed". He then made a conscious decision to share his wealth with the poor, the disadvantaged and the afflicted ones. Without understanding how this change happened his mission became "Never take more than what you give". He purchased a truck, equipped it with special handicap devices that compensated for his amputated toes. He visited food banks, homeless shelters and salvation army establishments in the Northeastern region and gave generously to all that were in need. He recognized God's love and knew that the doctor's prayer was answered. He gave of everything he had, even from crops he planted, always giving to others more than he took for himself.

Fascinating Life Cycle

Ronnie acquired skills in fishing and became particularly fascinated with the salmon life cycle. He observed the fully grown female salmons swimming through treacherous waterways from the ocean, going through dams, rocks and numerous to count natural obstacles. They seemed uncontrollably driven to reach river streams to lay their eggs. So many salmons never reach their destination. They are fished out, killed or eaten by bears, destroyed by rocks and dams. Then the school of new born salmons swim back from the river streams to the ocean to complete their circle of life. The salmon life cycle was captivating and it evoked a realistic awareness of the shortness of life. Ronnie was keenly cognizant that he would not live forever and that his life may end soon. He was not married, he had no children, and in a way similar to the salmons who perish during their treacherous journey from the oceans to the rivers. He felt an urgency to execute his last will and testimony.

Is This Denise?

On his way to his attorney office, the lively colors of Spring in a nearby park sparked his curiosity. He walked to the park and picked up a red rose that had fallen to the ground. Looking up he saw a lady with reddish golden hair. Could this be Denise? Hello she said. Ronnie looked up. It was not Denise, without any hesitation he gave her the red rose. She replied with a thank you and an angelic smile and asked what is your name?. Ronnie, with a quivering voice he answered, and what is yours? Lovejoy!! She asked if he was limping due to pain. He told her about the unfortunate avalanche accident and his lost dreams of being a runner. Tears dropped like rain, could not control her sobbing, she kissed him on the cheek, and asked if they could meet again. Ronnie was hesitant to agree since Lovejoy appeared much younger than him. As if she read his mind, she said, I know what you are thinking, no matter how old you are I care about you. She kissed him on the other cheek and felt as if he was touched by one of God 's loving angels.

A New Chapter Unfolds

As time passed they met many times in the same spot in the park. On a sunny day, Lovejoy confided deep secrets to Ronnie. She was an unwanted child and was, abused by her parents and grew up in various foster homes. She became pregnant at age 16 and underwent an abortion which made her infertile. She had 3 failed marriages due to her inability to conceive. Now at the age of 55, she has no family, no children and living on social welfare. On the day that he gave her the red rose she was contemplating suicide. Tears like rain trickled down Ronnie's cheeks and he could not control his sobbing. Lovejoy wanted to leave and run. She said she could not cope with his sobbing. Ronnie would not let go of her hands. That day they held hands for the first time. Ronnie realized he had not held any person's hand since the avalanche accident. Lovejoy confined that she has not held hands with anyone since her last divorce 10 years earlier. She then added that she has been homeless since then. Ronnie extended her an invitation to come live in the guest wing of his mansion. Without hesitation, she agreed, she felt safe, secure and spiritually fulfilled.

A Vision In The Midst Of A Thunder

Three years passed, Ronnie and Lovejoy enjoyed each others companionship and introduced themselves to others as having a platonic love relationship. One day Lovejoy was babysitting the neighbor's baby girl and was uncontrollably crying. She wished she could raise children that she could call her own. Ronnie felt her deep sorrow as if a sharp knife had pierced his heart. That evening it was raining. Thunder and lightning engulfed the mansion with brightness. Ronnie reflected that he too had a deeply felt longing to be called a "daddy". He had been demoralized with lost dreams of becoming an Olympic runner, and he had never contemplated ever having a family. The bright light surroundings created a vision. With all his given material possession and wealth, he could bring joy and fulfilment to hundreds and hundreds of needy children. He shared his vision with Lovejoy who with a sense of awe shared that she had an identical vision. Moments of silence passed. Coincidently a documentary appeared on the television set which was momentarily turned off during the lightning storm. The TV screen showed an adolescent girl pleading someone to come to a village in Africa. In that village, all unwed mothers were kept in a rundown facility and were forced to abort their unborn children.

Birth Of A Mission

Without the uttering of any word, Ronnie and Lovejoy hugged and the following week they flew to that village in Africa. Many unwed mothers who wished to keep their unborn children. They were told that there are no financial means to care for these mothers and their expected newborns. Ronnie returned back to his mansion, liquidated all his assets, sold his property and belongings and returned to the village. He lived in a small cottage and initiated a special trust to oversee all the needs and expenses of these mothers and their children. Lovejoy was chosen as his estate trustee and the sole recipient of inheritance. Joy, peace and multiple babies filled Ronnie's and Lovejoy's lives. Ronnie taught the villagers new ways to hunt, to fish and to grow crops, as well as raising family units. God's love was revealed to the village inhabitants, to the mothers and to the multiplying scores of newborn children. Over the following years, there were no unwed mothers. Engagement followed by festive weddings abounded. All the villagers prospered and they felt the presence of God in their midst.

Running to Heaven

One bright, crispy day, the village had planned with Lovejoy an extravagant, festive carnival to celebrate Ronnie's eighty fifth birthday. Although frail and weak, Ronnie felt young and healthy, strong and fit.

His soul seemed to have been seized by a divine power. He was listening to an inner voice, his parents encouraging whispers, and his coaches cheering shouts. He saw all his high school track and field trophies lining up on silver clouds. He heard distinct voices calling *Run Ronnie Run Run Ronnie Run*. He stood up, bended and got ready and, he ran, ran, ran until his last breath. His spirit was at last liberated to fly to the heavenly realms. He had a funeral that honored his life and it was filled with the joy and laughter usually reserved for birthday celebrations. Children, fathers, mothers, grandparents along with the entire village with its birds, its land and its ocean sang Run Ronnie Run. They sang good bye and farewell. Their voices were heavenly and angelic. His tombstone was placed on the highest hill surrounded by flowers and inscriptions from all the village inhabitants. Despite her immense grief Lovejoy carried the torch and lead the village in living a fulfilled earthly life with a spiritual link to the heavenly. With her gained wisdom, she helped the villagers to become economically self- sufficient, and with her practical shrewdness the village assets were multiplied by so many folds.

Farewell and Commencement

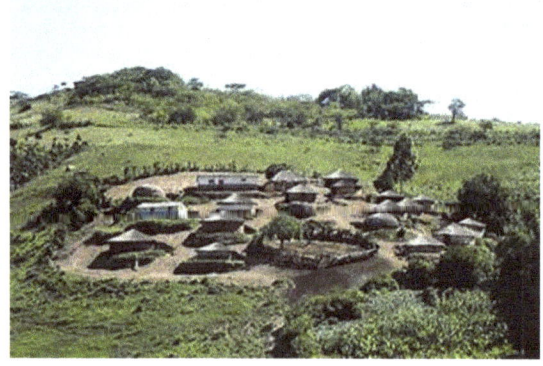

One day while holding a newborn baby girl Lovejoy kissed her, hugged her and caressed her tiny face. Lovejoy felt the joy of motherhood and gently sang to the baby girl "my baby my baby".

Lovejoy's spirit flew like a dove to the heavens while she was singing this lullaby. Her tombstone was placed next to Ronnie's. The children, their mothers, their fathers, and their grandparents sang their farewells and good byes all night long. The village and its inhabitants learned and applied the principles of God's true love, the values of generosity, and to "Never take more than what you give". Ronnie and Lovejoy victorious lives had brought joy, love, peace, hope, prosperity and a new dawn to this African village and hopefully to the whole surrounding world.

*Segments previously published in; Khouzam HR. Ronnie and Lovejoy :A Narrative of Giving and Remission of Suicidal Intentions. *Theranostics of Brain Disorder*. 1(2): 1-3, 2017.

TALE XII

*Social Phobia**

Be Still My Soul

Since her mid-teens, Geraldine had excessive fears of being in any social setting and concerns of being judged by others for being anxious, weak, or "nerdy". During conversation with others, her voice often trembled, and was labeled as a stutterer. In addition, she almost always experienced blushing in any public event. Although she graduated from high school with honors, the social anxiety and, specifically, the fears of being scrutinized by others, initially prevented her from pursuing her childhood dream of joining the institute of performing arts, following in the footsteps of her maternal grandmother who was a famous Soprano Opera singer.

Designing Jewelry

Geraldine's exceptional artistic talents in designing and making jewelry allowed her to be employed by a wealthy jeweler who hired her and let her work in a secluded area of the shop where she was completely sheltered from public contact. Geraldine adamantly rejected multiple suggestions from family members to consider medication as treatment for social anxiety (also known as social phobia); however, she was regularly receiving cognitive behavioral therapy including cognitive restructuring and exposure therapy. She was also involved in a self-help group with other individuals with social phobia. The group members met weekly to learn and practice social interactions. The combination of the therapy and group attendance along with the unconditional support she received from her parents and four siblings led to a decrease in the intensity of the social phobia.

Engaged to be Married

At the age of 20, and during a blind date Geraldine was introduced to Steve, a 22 year old young man. She instantly felt comfortable with Steve. Their interpersonal relationship grew and over the following nine months, they went to several public events together. As their relationship strengthened, Geraldine realized that her social anxiety was less disturbing. As a result of this improvement, which was also noticed by her family, she stopped attending the cognitive behavioral therapy sessions and withdrew from the self-help group.

By the age of 22, Geraldine continued to experience feelings of comfort and freedom from anxiety when she interacted in public settings. Steve had proposed to marry her, they were engaged, and they set their wedding date to coincide with her 23nd birthday celebration. In addition, she fulfilled her long-awaited dream when she was successfully accepted at the Institute of Performing Arts.

Here We Go Again

In the course of her first semester at the Institute; Geraldine was exposed to multiple novel situations and began to experience recurrence of symptoms of social phobia. These symptoms were manifested in trembling hands, inarticulate voice which resembled stuttering, increased blushing, hyperventilation, and sweating. Embarrassed by the quality of her voice, which is a necessary requirement for singing. She began to avoid interacting with her classmates and withdraw from several mandated singing practices. She felt ashamed, embarrassed, and her school performances markedly deteriorated and was eventually placed on probation with a looming possibility of being expelled from the Institute of Performing Arts. The anticipation of her wedding ceremony provoked intense feelings of social anxiety and she contemplated the prospect of breaking her engagement to Steve.

No Resolution In Site

Geraldine's family along with Steve showered her with love, care and emotional support and encouraged her to resume cognitive therapy and attendance of the self-help group. She then experienced heart palpitation, gastrointestinal discomfort, muscle tension, and confusion. These symptoms were frequent and severely intense and led to an indefinite postponement of the wedding. She stopped attending the therapy and the group sessions and rejected all suggestions to pursue medications treatment for social phobia.

Given her religious upbringing, during a particular religious event, with persuasion and relentless encouragement, Geraldine accompanied her youngest sister to her church choir performance. The choir sang the hymn, Be Still, My Soul with words by von Schlegel (1752) inspired from Psalm 46: 10 with the tune from "Finlandia" by Sibelius (1899):

Be Still My Soul

Be still, my soul; the Lord is on thy side;
Bear patiently the cross of grief or pain;
Leave to thy God to order and provide;
In every change He faithful will remain.
Be still, my soul: thy best, thy heav'nly Friend
Thro' thorny ways leads to a joyful end.
Be still, my soul: thy God doth undertake
To guide the future as He has the past.
Thy hope, thy confidence let nothing shake;
All now mysterious shall be bright at last.
Be still, my soul: the waves and wind still know
His voice who ruled them while he dwelt below.
Be still, my soul: the hour is hast'ning on
When we shall be forevr with the Lord,
When disappointment, grief, and fear are gone.
Sorrow forgot, love's purest joys restored.

Be still, my soul: when changes and tears are past,
All safe and blessed we shall meet at last.

Liberated at Last

Geraldine was surprised to notice the profound effects that the hymn and the music had on evoking and renewing her religious beliefs. She made a determined decision to rely on these beliefs as a mean of deliverance from her social anxiety. She began the process of memorizing *Be Still My Soul* by listening to it several times daily until she repeated it perfectly and sang its tune with her non quivering Opera worthy voice. Over the ensuing 6 weeks, Geraldine noticed that, whenever she experienced social phobia, she sang the hymn and would instantly experience remission of heart palpitations, gastrointestinal discomfort, muscle tension, and mental confusion. Initially, Geraldine's family and her fiancé Steve doubted her report of improvement and attributed it to her wishful thinking. Over the ensuing 4 months, the social phobia symptoms constantly and predictably subsided whenever Geraldine sang *Be Still My Soul* hymn.

With her persistence dedication to singing the hymn, her voice gained more perfection in its operatic quality and in its strength.

An Accomplished Opera Singer

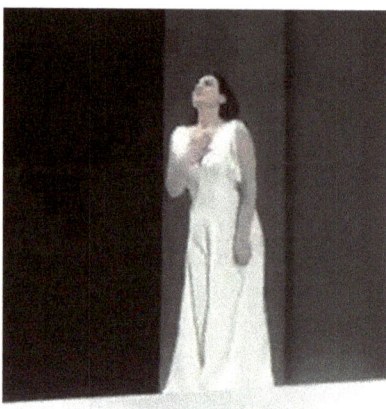

Subsequently Geraldine was accepted for readmission to the Institute of Performing Arts and qualified for the Soprano role and sang in the Institute performance of the Opera *Othello*. Her mother called her 3 sisters who were living in other states to exert all their efforts for an impromptu visit so they could attend the 5th and last Institute performance of *Othello*.

They all came and listened to their niece outstanding Soprano voice which reignited the cherished memories of their mother's singing career. They reaffirmed the great similarity between Geraldine and her grandmother unique singing style. They wished that their mother was still around to witness her granddaughter preservation of her singing legacy.

Special Wedding

Geraldine continued to excel in her performing arts courses. She confidently reset her wedding date on Steve 26th birthday. That date was an endeared occasion for Steve's family, since it coincided with the date of his parents gaining public recognition for their volunteer work with the Salvation Army. The wedding ceremony did not evoke any fears or anxiety. It was a unique and special wedding because Geraldine sang her own wedding songs and with her Operatic voice and received standing ovation from the wedding guests when she sang *Be Still My Soul*

Enduring Reliance

Geraldine and Steve had 3 daughters, all were inclined to sing, their house hold was a lively and joyful home. Geraldine did experience episodic recurrence of social anxiety. They were usually mild and short lived. She frequently conveyed to Steve and to her daughters that singing the hymn *Be Still My Soul*, did cement her total reliance on God's provision of calm and freedom from social anxiety. She convincedly believe that the stillness of her soul brought on the relief from the disabling effects of social phobia. Her upbringing in a religious home also contributed to her acceptance of God's ever presence in every aspect of her life. She marveled at the empowering and enduring effects of the hymn *Be Still My Soul*, which inspired her, mobilized her inner resources and liberated her from social phobia.

*Segments previously published in; Khouzam HR, Ghaffori B, Nichols EAE. Use of a religious hymn in remission of symptoms of social phobia (social anxiety disorder): A case study. *Psychological Reports* 96:411-421, 2005.

TALE XIII

*Acceptance Commitment Therapy**
The Lord's Prayer

Sion is a 22 year-old single male Samoan wrestler who had childhood-onset post traumatic stress disorder (PTSD) related to being cruelly abused emotionally and physically by his stepfather. Reportedly his stepfather, the proprietor of his constant abuse, used to put hot frying pans over his head, lock him for several days in a closet with only water to drink, not allowing him to use the bathroom and on many occasions threatening to burn him while hanging from a tree. When he was 6 years old, the stepfather was charged with endangering of a life of a minor and was sentenced to a long term imprisonment. Then the patient's mother surrendered her parental rights due to inability to raise him. He was adopted by a Samoan couple who lived in Australia and who devoted their life to nurturing him and to providing for all of his emotional, educational, social and physical needs.

Effects of a Cruel Up-Bringing

Despite the safety of his new environment, Sion continued to experience PTSD symptoms that included recurrent nightmares, marked anxiety with hypervigilance, and persistent avoidance of males, especially those who had a similar voice tone or resembled his stepfather. He was evaluated by a child psychiatrist, who diagnosed him with childhood-onset PTSD. His adoptive parents attended several supportive psychotherapy sessions and exerted dedicated efforts to help him separate himself from the traumatic events and from the victim role. His adoptive mother who had a background as a social worker in maternal and child health; implemented interventions at home and the immediate neighborhood environments that were aimed on reducing risks of exposure to triggers of physical or emotional abuse.

State Of The Art Interventions

These interventions included the ongoing provision of personal support, socialization, development of coping skills and strengthening of self-esteem. Constant efforts were implemented and practiced with the goal of conveying a clear message of being valued as an essential member of a family that shared encouraging values, communicated openly, and provided care, love and emotional closeness. The beneficial effects of these interventions were also supported and validated by the child psychiatrist and the pediatrician who followed Sion annually for his regular medical check-up and psychiatry follow-up. These interventions seemed to have positive effects, and between the ages of 6 and 13 years Sion did not reports PTSD symptoms of avoidance, hypervigilance, or mood irregularities. That improvement was observed by his parents and confirmed by his child psychiatrist and pediatrician feedbacks. Sion seemed to have developed trusting relationships with his adoptive father and two male teachers. As he continued to experience feelings of safety, and a sustained remission of frightening nightmares.

Successful in School

Sion parents out of respect of their heritage enrolled Sion in a private Catholic school. He seemed to have emotionally flourished and excelled in academics, in singing and in sports. He was chosen on numerous special religious events to sing one of his favorite pieces, "*The Lord's Prayer*". His parents, his neighbors, and classmates always remarked that the themes and the melody of singing the *Lord's Prayer* had calming and peaceful effects on his general demeanor. Although his parents were not practicing Catholics, he asked them if he could become a Catholic and if he could have a first communion ceremony with his classmates and they agreed.

Fencing Championship

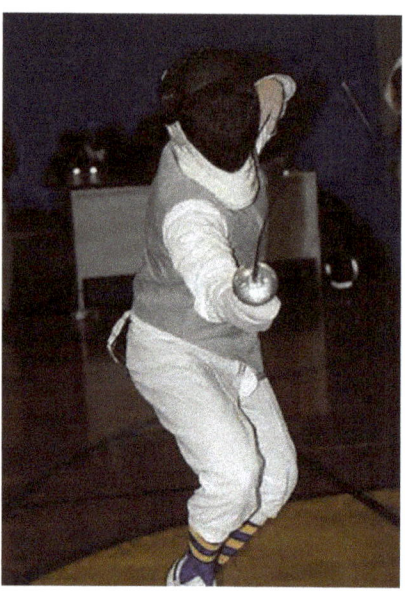

By the age of 17, Sion was considered one of the best school athletes in several sports and particularly in fencing. During a championship fencing dual match, one of the referees drew his attention to his untied shoe laces. Suddenly and unexpectedly, he turned around and tried to stab the referee's chest with his fencing sabre. Fortunately the referee was able to evade this sudden move. Sion was restrained and escorted to the locker room where he kept shouting, "I will kill him, and I will kill him." He was suspended from fencing and from school attendance. His parents sought a psychiatric evaluation, which confirmed that this episode of trying to kill the referee was triggered by the referee's tone of voice, which had similar qualities to his abusive stepfather's voice. He then began to experience no remitting episodes of anger, anxiety, hypervigilance, mood liability, and frightening nightmares. His parents were not comfortable with the notion of giving him medications for these symptoms, and agreed with the school psychologist recommendation of referral to individual psychotherapy.

Response to Therapy

Based on his self-report, Sion felt that therapy helped in counteracting the effects of the recurrent distressing feelings. These feelings were apparently the result of his remembrance of his stepfather abusive actions. Furthermore his parents reported a great sense of relief noting the de-escalation of anxiety, anger, hypervigilance, and mood lability. He also reported a remission of the frightening nightmares. Sion attributed his improvement to the practicing of the techniques that he learned during his therapy. He credited his general emotional wellbeing to the tremendous support he received from his parents, his classmates, and his teachers. Despite his school suspension, his teachers, and coaches kept in touch with him and his parents. He took it upon himself to personally apologize to the referee who he had tried to hurt and agreed as an act of restitution to complete a 7-weeks period of serving as a volunteer orderly in a community senior citizen center.

Wrestling

He found the elderly residents to be caring and nurturing. His parents rejoiced when they heard him say, "After all, there are good people in this world." His school suspension was reversed but he was not allowed to resume fencing. He shifted his interest to featherweight wrestling and became a member of the school wrestling team. At the age of 18 as a result of his academic and sports excellence, he earned a scholarship and enrolled in the University with an elective in an advanced photography course.

He continued to excel academically and in wrestling and at the age of 21 he was chosen to join the team that was competing in the Annual National Featherweight Wrestling Universities Championship.

Prior to a round of wrestling, a Samoan wrestler came toward him to greet him and attempted to shake his hand. He responded by loudly screaming, "Get away from me, I mean it, I will break your neck and kill you." That wrestler stature and walking pattern reminded him of his abusive stepfather. He was escorted off the hall and was later admitted to an acute care psychiatric unit due to his expression of homicidal intentions toward the Samoan wrestler. He was also experiencing recurrence of PTSD symptoms.

Another Hospital Admission

Given the severity and intensity of his PTSD symptoms, the treatment team recommended the use of an antidepressant medication in combination with psychotherapy. Sion adamantly refused all suggested medications but agreed to receive Acceptance Commitment Therapy (ACT); a behaviorally based therapy that is especially designed to target and reduce experiential avoidance and cognitive entanglement while encouraging the pursuit of behavioral changes that correspond with personal values. The main objective in ACT was to increase Sion's psychological flexibility. Psychological flexibility involves contacting the present moment, while remaining behaviorally committed to living a principled life, even when the mind advises otherwise. Sion showed a good response during his first 2 sessions of ACT. He was evaluated by his treatment team and was deemed safe to be discharged from the hospital.

What's Next?

Following his hospital discharge Sion was transferred to a residential respite care facility for ongoing stabilization and continuation of ACT. He completed 22 additional weekly sessions of ACT and regained his calm. He recognized his dangerous mistake of threatening to kill the Samoan wrestler just because he reminded him of his abusive stepfather. He was thankful due to the beneficial effects of ACT in decreasing the PTSD symptoms of intrusive thoughts, avoidant behaviors, and alterations in his perception of individuals who remind him of his abusive stepfather. Unfortunately these positive emotional responses evaporated quickly when a visitor to the residential respite care facility accidently run into him in the reception area. Without any warning signs, Sion wrestled the visitor and knocked him to the ground and attempted to break his neck. Reportedly that visitor's appearance was similar to his abusive stepfather.

Middle School Singing Quartet

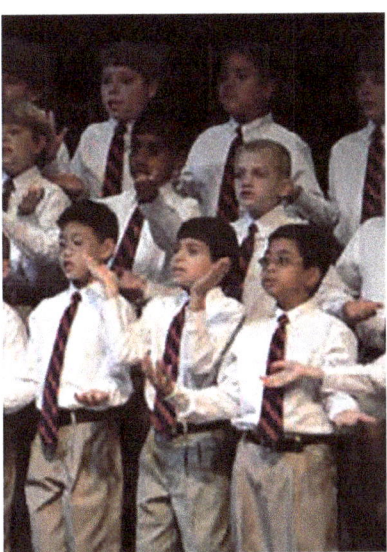

Swiftly and decisively, the staff intervened and rescued the visitor from Sion's hand grips. He became aggressive and combative and could not be retrained. At this particular moment a middle school singing quartet arrived for their weekly visit to the respite care facility. On Thursdays every week, this group of young boys would come to sing various songs to the respite care residents. On that particular Thursday they were fulfilling a resident request to sing the *Lord's Prayer*. Upon hearing their voices; Sion immediately stopped combating the staff. He quietly sat on the ground and joined in singing the *Lord's Prayer*.

A Reprise

Sion mind traveled back to his younger years when he attended the Catholic school and chosen on numerous special religious events to sing one of his favorite pieces, *"The Lord's Prayer"*. Following the completion of the prayer, Sion confined to his treatment team that ACT played a valuable role in reinforcing the section of the *The Lord's Prayer* that emphasizes "**Forgive us our debts, as we also have forgiven our debtors**". He declared with sincerity that his long held intentions to harm his stepfather have forever vanished. He confirmed that he has developed a sense of inner peace and consciously decided to forgive his abusive stepfather. His homicidal urges have permanently disappeared not only toward his childhood abuser, but for all the individuals who resembled his abusing stepfather. Sion resumed attending the University and returned back to practice featherweight wrestling with his team. He was confident that his wrestling team will for sure win their upcoming tournament and that he will eventually graduate with honors and accolades.

*Segments previously published in; Khouzam HR, Mathew JJ, Nile LM, Galvez SR. Case Study of Acceptance Commitment Therapy for Childhood Onset Posttraumatic Stress Disorder: A Patient's Unique Use of the Lord's Prayer. *J Trauma Stress Disor Treat*. 5:1, 2016.

TALE XIV

Inseparable Friends

The Legacy of an Architect and a Photographer

From Kindergarten through high school Alice and Renata were inseparable friends. They shared a dream that one day together they will travel across the world. Going to college temporary widened their physical proximity. Graduate school reunited them back. Alice pursued photography and Renata chose architecture. They enrolled in the School of the Art Institute of Chicago.

Reviving the Dream

It took a while for Alice and Renata to catch up. During their 4 years of separation while attending college their dream of traveling the globe was placed on the back burner. As they rekindled their inseparable bond their dream was reborn. They thought that may be in 2 or a maximum of 3 years they will complete graduate school and earnestly plan their long awaiting travel.

Graduate Studies

Alice studied travel photography which involved the documentation of various landscapes, cultures, customs, history and people. Her courses of study included practical experiences and travelling to many countries. Renata courses in architecture were arduous and thought provoking. Due to their outstanding performances they graduated in 2 years. Both had to take a 3 months practicum course after graduation. They renewed their passports to get ready to travel across the world in about 3 months.

Surfing in South Africa

Alice had an invitation from a classmate who was from South Africa to come visit her and her parents who lived in Cape Town. During her visit she spent time taking spectacular photograph of the waterfront with its breathtaking beaches. One day, her classmate brother invited her to come surf on Sandy Bay Beach. Although she did not know how to surf, she tremendously enjoyed the experience and wanted to surf again. On the fourth day of surfing, she noticed another surfer struggling to get on his board. She reached out to hold him up. Unexpectedly a colossal 40 ft high wave knocked her under the surfing board and she could not rise up above the wave. She drowned !!!

Getting Rid of the Passport

Renata was devasted, her best and inseparable friend is gone. They will not fulfill their childhood dream of traveling across the world. Anger and frustration overwhelmed Renata and she wanted to rip her passport or burn it. Her neighbor intervened. She reminded Renata of the memorial service which was planned for Alice in Cape Town and she needed her passport to travel to South Africa.

A Shanty Town

Following Alice heart wrenching memorial service, Renata was struck by the appearance of the shanty town of Khayelitsha. Alice classmate recalled hearing her saying that if Renata was visiting, she would have designed an architectural plan to change the shanty town precarious haphazard establishments into real livable homes with social and civic services. Renata pondered if she could fulfill Alice vision of changing the shanty town of Khayelitsha.

Hong Kong

Renata returned home from South Africa with a heavy heart that was riddled with grief and sadness. She has forever lost her inseparable friend Alice. Four years passed, one day while designing a mansion for a wealthy entrepreneur who resided in Florida, she noticed that he had an album of photographs of shanty towns in Hong Kong. These towns were infringing on the borders of the high rise buildings and skyscrapers. City planners were concerned about the economic ramification of these shanty towns. Non-governmental organizations with strong ties with the entrepreneur had set in motion an ambitious plan of transforming the shanty towns of Hong Kong into modern cities. The plan included building adequate infrastructure, implementing proper sanitation, securing a safe water supply and street drainage, and establishing an electricity grid.

South Africa

Renata approached the wealthy entrepreneur Richard. She showed him the photographs that she took of the shanty town of Khayelitsha in Cape Town, South Africa. He remained silent and then nodded his head and mentioned that he is not familiar with the laws that govern South Africa construction codes and regulations but promised to consider that project. In the meantime Renata opened a small box that Alice parents had given her. It had memorabilia, letters, and many items of their shared childhood and adulthood years. One of these items was Alice passport. Renata then recalled the common dream of traveling across the world. Now without Alice the dream will never be realized. Once again she seriously considered getting rid of her own passport.

The Development of Khayelitsha

Richard had good news. South Africa construction codes had a provision for allowing international organizations to build and improve existing substandard structures including those in shanty towns. He was planning a large scale development for Khayelitsha in Cape Town, South Africa. He asked Renata to join the team that was assigned to that unprecedented project. Renata then realized that she had to keep her passport to travel back to South Africa.

Architectural Designs

Renata asked Alice parents if they had any sample of their daughter's traveling photographs. They had kept all of them to hold and to cherish her life's legacy. A year passed and a square mile of the shanty town of Khayelitsha in Cape Town, South Africa, was completely demolished and rebuilt into new living quarters. It resembled a modern city with paved roads, a beautiful park with a children playground, a row of neat apartments with electricity, running water and sanitary sewers. An inauguration event was organized. In the presence of the Mayor of Cape Town and many dignitaries, Renata and Alice parents were the honorary guests of the first Khayelitsha ribbon cutting ceremony. In Khayelitsha new town center a memorial garden was planted with a marble stone inscription "In Honor of Alice a Visionary Photographer -Although not in our Midst, she will forever Reside in our Hearts"

Wedding Invitation

Renata felt sad, her inseparable friend Alice although remembered, revered and honored, she is not around. The dream of traveling around the world need to be vanished. Getting rid of her passport will assure the permanent extinction of that dream. She was invited to attend her niece wedding in Mexico. She was not in the mood to be in a festive and happy occasion. She was just going to send her niece a gift without attending the wedding ceremony and reception. Renata's mother encouraged her to attend the wedding to see many of her relatives that she has not kept contact with for many years and to accompany her grandparents who wish to visit Mexico to see and spend time with their relatives. Renata's parents and siblings had flown earlier to Mexico and could not find seats on their flight for the grandparents.

Childhood Memories

Renata was born in Mexico, in the city of Guadalajara. Her parents and her grandparents moved to the US when she was 9 months old. Her maternal grandparents lived in the same household and helped raise her. Renata's parents were busy working to provide for their parents and their 6 children. The grandparents stayed with the family until Renata's mother left her job as a hotel house keeper, when Renata's father found a permanent job in construction and was able to provide for his family. Renata remembered with fondness the cherished time she spent teaching English to her grandparents. They were very attentive to her instructions, however they were not able to master speaking in English. So Renata booked a flight to Mexico to attend her niece wedding and to accompany her grandparents who were on the same flight. She was a great asset to her grandparents, facilitating and coordinating their travel documents and aiding with translation and in helping them complete custom and border security forms.

Guadalajara

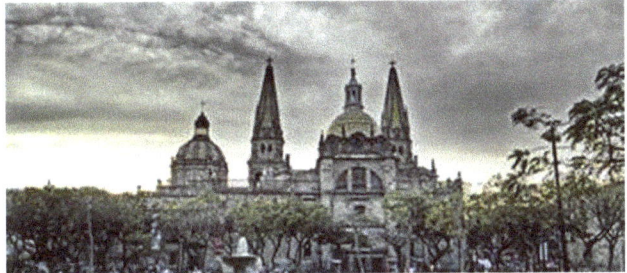

During the wedding reception, Renata sat next to her grandmother who asked her if she could take some time off her work as an architect to accompany her and her grandfather to visit Guadalajara. Renata's grandparents Miguel and Elena, kissed the ground when their plane landed in Guadalajara. An emotional scene that brought tears even to some bystanders. It was a 3 weeks reunion between Miguel and Elena with relatives and friends whom they have not seen for nearly half a decade. They also visited Isabella the midwife that delivered Renata. Isabella recalled that Renata was born with her eyes opened and a big smile. She then asked if she could seek her assistance in teaching English to the newly trained midwives who were longing to learn the English language so they could read modern English textbooks that were not yet translated in Spanish.

Renata promised to think about that proposition after she return home and consult with her architecture firm.

An Irresistible Offer

Richard the wealthy entrepreneur asked Renata if she could relocate to Florida. He offered her a 3 years contract to design building projects of transforming the shanty towns in Hong Kong to modern cities. She could not resist his proposed generous salary. With the marked increase in her annual income, Renata was able to afford travelling twice a year to Guadalajara where she stayed for a month to teach English to the midwives who under Isabelle leadership opened a school of midwifery. The school graduated competent and compassionate midwives who improved the prenatal care of pregnant mothers and had a positive impact on delivering healthy babies.

Happily Married

Richard proposed to Renata, she accepted and they married. Renata travelled across the world accompanying Richard on his many building projects. She always carried with her Alice passport as if they were travelling together. Alice legacy as a photographer never faded with the ongoing renovation of Khayelitsha in South Africa. A new legacy was also born with the modernization and rebuilding of shanty towns worldwide.

Post-Script

The legacy of the inseparable friends Alice and Renata started with a dream to travel across the world and left unforgettable marks of renovation of Khayelitsha in South Africa and shanty towns worldwide. A passport that was at the verge of being destroyed, was used to travel across the globe and going twice a year for many years to the city of Guadalajara in Mexico to teach English to midwives. Young midwives had the opportunity to learn English and to read and practice all the modern advances in delivering healthy babies. Although not physically present, Alice soul was front and center in Renata heart and mind. With each new travel, Renata used her passport along with Alice's which she has kept in her shirt pocket sewed close to her heart.

TALE XV

*Bulimia Nervosa**
Jumping and Landing

Bulimia nervosa (BN) is an eating disorder which is characterized by frequent episodes of binge eating followed by certain ritualist behaviors such as inducing vomiting, using laxatives, fasting, and exercising excessively to prevent gaining weight. Individuals with BN are helpless and unable to control their excessive eating. They are usually overburdened with feeling of guilt and sadness due to their uncontrolled eating habits

Sneak to Eat

Dedra a 33-year-old female, developed BN, at the age of 17. Her over eating episodes started following each dinner. She would ask her parents to be excused from the dining room to complete her homework and instead she will consume large quantity of food that she stored in a large ice cooler, hidden in her closet under several items of clothing. She would usually eat 2 medium size boxes of chocolate cookies, a large bag of potato ships, a medium size box of cheese crackers, 3 bowls of cereal with 2 cups of chocolate milk, and a bag of M &M. Following each episode of food consumption she would immediately force herself to vomit.

No more Binging

Sandra used most of her weekly allowance and the money she earned from babysitting in food purchases, her parents became suspicious about the possibility of alcohol or drug use, however one of her close friends who accidently discovered the ice cooler informed her parents. The parents understood their daughter's eating struggles since her maternal aunt had suffered from binge eating during her adolescence. The school psychologist recommended cognitive behavioral therapy (CBT) as an intervention for BN. Sandra successfully completed 12 weeks of CBT and experienced a remission of BN.

Looking Like A Balloon

For no apparent reason when she was 21 years old, Sandra resumed the nightly episodes of binge eating consuming 3 peanut jelly sandwiches, 2 cartons of chocolate milk, a box of cheese crackers, a tub of tapioca rice pudding and a medium size jar of strawberry jam followed by forced vomiting. At the time she was an 8 th grade teacher and had many children in her classroom who were overweight, she was extremely frightened by the thought of gaining extra-weight as the children. She began to use laxatives, joined a physical fitness club and exercised on a daily basis in an effort to control her weight. She came to realize that she looked like an overinflated balloon.

Where Do I Go

Sandra was visiting London with her friend, another teacher at their same school. During that time there was a 2019 performance of the 1967 musical Hair. One of the song that touched her was "Where do I go"

Where do I go
   Follow the river
      Where do I go
         Follow the gulls

Where is the something
   Where is the someone
      That tells me why I live and die

Where do I go
    Follow the children
        Where do I go
            Follow their smiles

Is there an answer
    In their sweet faces
        That tells me why I live and die

Reflecting on these special lyrics, she thought about her classroom's overweight children. She could hardly wait to return back home. Instead of rejecting the children who were overweight, Sandra longed to look into their sweet faces and to follow their smiles.

Getting Involved

On the first day of school, Sandra was eager to look at the overweight children from a different perspective. She asked the school principal if she could send a letter to the children parents inviting them to initiate an after school program of creative activities. The purpose of the program was to design fun physical activities that distract the children from using comfort food. Without referring to it as a weight loss program. Many of the parents were receptive and the "Jump high and safely land " initiative was created.

Jump High and Safely Land

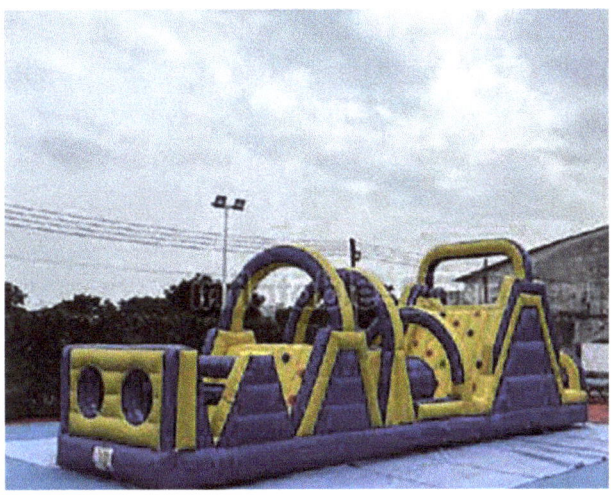

Donations of plastic ladders, and LEGO construction pieces were elicited from toys and department stores. Large cushioned floor mattresses were also bought at discount prices through social media advertisements. Over a 3 weeks period, Sandra along with the children and their parents constructed an easily assembled and disassembled gigantic LEGO fortress that used ladders to reach its highest elevation. Children will safely climb the ladders then jump in the air to land on the ground mattresses.

Rousing Success

The jumping and landing exercises were a big hit. Sandra, the children, the parents and the school administrators promoted it as a new sporting event. The overweight children along with Sandra shed their extra weight without their conscious awareness. Joyful hearts and healthier bodies filled the school hallways. Children abandoned their comfort food habits. Every new school year became an opportunity for Sandra to introduce the "Jump high and safely land " to the overweight children.

Following the Children

It began with a loss of control over excessive eating leading to self-induced vomiting to lose the gained weight. Inspiration then was born from the musical Hair with its unique song "where do I go" foretelling about the children smiles and their sweet faces. Creativity soon followed by jumping and landing using ladders and LEGO structures. Peeling off extra weight in the midst of rejoicing. Guilt, shame and Sandra's faulty self- image of being an overinflated balloon, were all forever gone.

. * Segments previously published in; Khouzam HR. The combination of Levomilnacipran, Cognitive behavior therapy and Christian based self–help group in the treatment of bulimia nervosa: A case report. Clinical and Experimental Psychology. 2:3, 2016.

TALE XVI

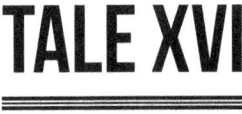

Shortened life

Heavenly Sisterhood Bond

Amber and Dave have been married for 3 years and yearning to have a baby. After so many in-vitro fertilization trials a beautiful healthy baby girl Angel was born. She was the love of their life. Angel was cheerful and calm. At the age 9 months she slept through the night giving her parents the gift of restful and refreshing sleep. She began speaking with complete sentences at the age of 13 months. As a precious and unique daughter, Amber and Dave devoted all their time and energy to care and to love her. They halted their activities of going to dinner with friends and ballroom dancing. Their parents were concerned about their burnout and on many occasions they offered to babysit Angel, to no avail.

New Neighbors

Angel in now 2 years old, vivacious, adorable and beautiful. It is Amber and Dave 5th wedding anniversary. A family of a husband and wife and their 2 daughters recently bought the house across the street. Vanessa the 19 years old daughter is an experienced babysitter with many certificates of appreciation, that she received from many parents when she lived in Ohio.

Babysitter

With their parents, persuasion and despite their trepidation they asked Vanessa if she could babysit Angel while they go out to dinner to celebrate their 5th wedding anniversary. Hoping that she would either refuse or that Angel would not warm up to a stranger. Surprise, surprise, Vanessa was free that night and Angel instantly welcomed her and showed her special collection of Barbie dolls.

It was indeed a delightful evening and a delicious dinner which revived their honeymoon memories. In the meantime Angel and Vanessa created imaginative Barbie Dolls happy ending fairy tales. Exhausted from almost 4 hours of non- interrupted play, they fell asleep on the bedroom floor. Earlier Vanessa had warmed up a precooked dinner meal, and in the midst of the fun play time, she forgot to turn the stove off.

Kitchen on Fire

Kitchen towels fell, caught flames, fire ignited, fumes spread, firefighters summoned to the scene. Vanessa was revived, Angel died from smoke inhalation.

Agony, broken hearts, unshakable grief. Vanessa and her parents could not face the indescribable tragedy, they placed their home on a quick sale and returned back to Ohio. Amber and Dave parents with their unspeakable sadness blamed themselves for pressuring their children to go to dinner on that tragic evening. Amber succumbed to insurmountable depression and Dave was constantly contemplating suicide as the only mean to end his emotional suffering.

Earthquake in Haiti

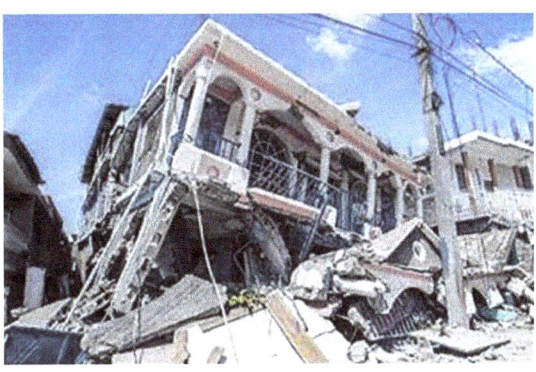

In January of 2010, a catastrophic earthquake struck Haiti, which was followed by at least 52 aftershock. Hundred thousands of lives perished. Thousands of buildings collapsed and surviving Haitians were surrounded by unimaginable devastation. Many countries responded to appeals for humanitarian aid, pledging funds and dispatching rescue and medical teams, engineers and support personnel. The most-watched telethon in history called "Hope for Haiti Now, " was aired encouraging volunteers from all walk of life to join in the efforts of reconstructing the country.

A Call to Serve

After 2 years of grief and void and with her background in nursing Amber felt an inner calling to join a medical organization that was recruiting volunteers to help in Haiti. Dave was still devastated, devoid of living and very depressed. As a constructor, his skills were in high demand in Haiti. Amber begged Dave to join her on this humanitarian mission. He adamantly refused and warned her, that he may not be around when she returns.

Broken Arm

With a heavy heart and tearful eyes, Amber arrived to the shattered lives and demolished buildings of Haiti. In the midst of the rubbles in a makeshift field hospital many injured children were sleeping in tarp made structures. A noticeably small and poorly nourished little girl emerged with a broken left arm. Taken by her pleasant disposition, Amber immediately attended to her need and placed a cast around her tiny arm.

Need for Constructor Workers

Many constructor workers were showing sign of exhaustion and badly needed extra help. Amber for the first time since Angel death reached out to her in-laws and asked Dave father, Albert who was a contractor if he could come to Haiti. Her mother in- law Eugenia raised concerns given, Albert recent heart bypass surgery. Albert gathered all his inner strength and traveled with Eugenia for the first time in many years to their son's home. His front door was unlocked!

Prolonged Grief

Dave appeared to be in a stupor, surrounded by empty bottles of liquors and half eaten pizza slices. Awful smell of rottenness threw them both into a state of nausea and stomach sickness. Surprised by their sudden appearance, Dave jumped up and was about to choke them. He then regained his composure, apologized and with a loud and agonizing voice asked them to "get out". He burst into a crying fit, then shouting Albert and Eugenia names as the murderers of his Angel. He blamed them for encouraging the outing and the dining on his wedding anniversary. He cried out. If I was home that evening, Angel my one and only beloved daughter would have been alive.

Decision to Help

Albert and Eugenia cried with Dave through the night. Exhausted and drained they all fell asleep in his filthy living room. In the morning, storms of hungry flies woke them up by their buzzing wings. Eugenia told

Dave about his father recent heart surgery and that he was determined to travel to Haiti to help in its reconstruction. "No way Dad, he shouted, I will go, and you stay home".

Reconciliation

Dave in turn contacted his in-laws whom he has shunned away since they too did encourage the outing and the hiring of the baby sitter. Tom and Victoria initially thought that another tragedy had occurred. He reassured them and asked Tom if he would join him and travel to Haiti and help in the reconstruction efforts. If he agreed to do so, he would also have the chance to see his daughter Amber whom he has not seen for so long. Tom as an electrician by trade would be a valuable asset in installing electric wires and devices for the newly constructed homes and in the partially damaged structures.

Drawn to the Little Girl

A reunion of tears and sorrows between Amber, her husband Dave and her father Tom, ignited glimpses of hope. Once separated as if they were strangers now in a foreign land they are reunited with a humanitarian goal. Amber felt a sentimental attachment toward the tiny little girl with the broken arm. She inquired about her family, and was informed that her parents and 2 siblings did not survive the earthquake and she has no surviving relatives. Tom and Dave rolled up their sleeves and worked tirelessly every day. By night fall they were so exhausted to even converse before they fell asleep.

Her Name Is Anne

With every passing day, Amber grew closer and closer to the little tiny girl, her name was Anne. Deep in her heart she knew that nobody could replace her beloved Angel. Here is a lovely little girl without any family. What would happen to her? Where is she going to grow up? Who would care for her? She was in turmoil and felt as if she was caught in a whirlwind of conflicted emotions.

International Adoption

Amber approached her father Tom and asked him if he noticed Anne. To her surprise he did and he admitted that he was drawn to her. He wished he could hug her and shower her with kisses of endearment. A team of Red Cross workers were walking by and handing adoption applications. Tom took an application. He was extremely saddened. The application had big red colored letters forbidding International adoption.

Could She Be Their Daughter

Amber was engulfed by feelings of relief because Anne will not replace Angel and at the same time overwhelmed by sadness for missing the chance of becoming a mother of a lovely little girl. Tom confided his love for Anne to his son Dave. Dave admitted that he had the same sentiment. In the meantime Amber was feverishly studying Haiti's adoption laws. She found a clause related to an international adoption of a child if it is pursued by charitable or civic organizations.

There is a solution

Albert and Eugenia recalled that Vanessa the baby sitter had mentioned that her parents Bob and Liz were active Rotary Club administrators. They reached out to Dave their son and asked if he knew how to reach out to Bob and Liz. It was an arduous and complicated task. By all accounts and measures what ensued though surreal was miraculous.

Rotary Club

Bob and Liz petitioned their Rotary Club in Ohio to explore the possibility of petitioning the Haiti government for an international adoption. Despite insurmountable bureaucratic obstacles, the petition was favorably accepted. Tom, Dave and Amber wrapped up their 7 months of volunteer work in Haiti which earned them a special commendation and an expediated adoption. Bob, and Liz with their daughter Vanessa arrived to Haiti and along with Amber, Tom and Dave flew back to the US with Anne. On their arrival they were welcomed by Albert and Eugenia, along with Amber's mother Victoria and so many to count friends and relatives of Vanessa and her parents extended family.

Miracle in the Making

The many years of emotional, heartaches, resentment and prolonged grief over the tragic loss of Angel created a chasm of despair between all the people who loved her. Anne a child without parents or relatives seemed to have been destined to survive the Haiti devastating earthquake to mend the drift and reunite caring people around her, their new found miracle.

The Birth of an Agency

The Angel Adoption Agency International (AAAI) was born with its founding members Dave, Amber, Albert, Eugenia, Tom, Victoria, Bob, Liz and Vanessa. The purpose of AAAI was to raise funds that would facilitate the adoption of orphans from around the world. An agency or individual licensed for international adoptions would usually charges $20, 000 to $50, 000 for their international adoption services. The AAAI raised funds were given to prospective adopting parents who were approved by the existing adoption agencies but could not afford that relatively high cost.

International Law

Years marched on and Anne grown to become a bright and caring young lady. She graduated with a cum laude doctorate in international law. She played a significant role in improving and modernizing international adoption laws. The AAAI founding members assigned her as the sole trustee of their adoption agency. Under her dedicated efforts and tireless commitment hundreds of orphans were brought from across the globe to join their adoptive parents all over the USA. In a commencement address to a class of International Law Graduates, Anne recalled with teary eyes and a heart full of love an assignment she had in grade school.

Family Tree

The assignment was about drawing her family tree beginning with her great grandparents and ending with her and her siblings. Although she loved and dearly cherished her adoptive parents and grandparents, she could not draw the expected traditional family tree. Anne instead drew a straight tree trunk with golden rather than green color. She had a small portrait of herself at the bottom of the golden tree trunk. The top of the tree trunk reached the clouds and on one of the clouds sat a little girl with two tiny wings with a name inscription "my beloved sister Angel." That commencement address aroused 15 minutes of standing ovation and was reported in several newspaper headlines. The grade school family tree assignment at the time was kept in a uniquely created display frame at the grade school principal office.

Remembrance

The loss of so many lives due to the earthquake in Haiti and the shortened life of a beloved daughter in the US were disastrous and tragic events. Out of the rubbles of a destroyed building in Haiti, a little girl Anne emerged. The families that were shattered by the death of their beloved Angel were reunited with unconditional and immense love toward Anne. Anne fostered and sustained an international agency that allowed parents to adopt orphans from all across the globe. Although they never met, Anne created an enduring legacy honoring her sister Angel and all those who were grieved by her early departure from their world.

TALE XVII

Schizophrenia
Beware of Marijuana

Patients with schizophrenia usually receives antipsychotic medications for stabilization of their psychotic symptoms. Some of these symptoms include paranoid delusions and auditory hallucinations. Some of the patients receive long acting injectable antipsychotics usually given every month or every 3 months or even at longer intervals.

Treatment

In a community mental health center there were 2 patients who were diagnosed with schizophrenia and were receiving monthly injection of antipsychotic medications. The medications prevented the recurrence of psychotic symptoms. The 2 patients developed adverse effects to the antipsychotic medications that included excessive weight gain, metabolic syndrome and type 2 diabetes. Additionally the medications slowed them down due to lethargy and fatigue.

Disability Income

The 2 patients felt the beneficial effects of the antipsychotic medications and despite the adverse effects consented to receive them indefinitely. Due to their inability to sustain employment. The 2 patients received social security disability income that allowed them to acquire adequate food and shelter.

Severity of an Illness

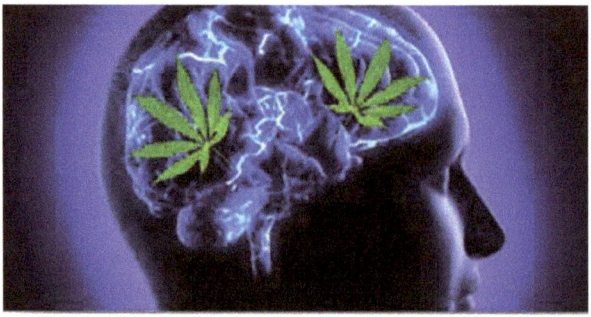

Marijuana and schizophrenia are serious mental disorders that can profoundly impact people's lives. Many people who use marijuana may not be able to stop using despite its negative consequences on their lives. Schizophrenia is a serious mental illness that affects how a person thinks, feels, and behaves. People with schizophrenia often seem to have lost touch with reality, and the symptoms of schizophrenia can make it difficult to participate in usual everyday activities. However, effective treatments are available for both marijuana use and schizophrenia.

New Research ＊

Many researchers found strong evidence of an association between marijuana use and schizophrenia among men and women, though the association is much stronger among young men. Statistical analysis have estimated that as many as 30% of cases of schizophrenia among men aged 21 30 might have been prevented by averting marijuana use.

Clinical Intervention

Although not everyone who use marijuana would develop schizophrenia and not everyone who has schizophrenia used marijuana. The 2 patients who were receiving antipsychotic medications, had used marijuana during their teen and adolescent years. It is not clear yet if people who developed schizophrenia due to marijuana use could achieve recovery if they sustain extended periods of abstinence from marijuana use and hopefully would lead a functional and productive life as a result of a remission of the symptoms of schizophrenia.

Response to Treatment

The 2 patients who were receiving long acting injectable antipsychotic medications have not used marijuana for more than 2 years. They were diagnosed with schizophrenia and their psychotic symptoms of paranoia, auditory hallucinations and disorganized thinking subsided as a result of treatment with the antipsychotic medications.

Dilemma

Is it possible that the marijuana use caused the development of schizophrenia? Is it also possible that without marijuana use these 2 patients will not have schizophrenia? Would stopping the antipsychotic medications lead to recurrence of psychosis or result in improved alertness and daily level of functioning?

Daring Decision

Their names are Ben and Ahmad. They want to be productive members of their society. They feel confident in their ability to abstain from marijuana use. They asked to be taken off the antipsychotic medications. Their decisions was supported and encouraged.

A Piano Player

Ben was 22 years old and growing up he loved to play the piano. The last time he touched his grandmother grand piano was on Christmas eve. He was 15 years old and played the song Silent Night. Years of marijuana use seemed to have erased his yearning and his love of music. He was taken off the antipsychotic medication. Three months passed and his love for playing the piano was rekindled. He volunteered to join his city orchestra. During a Spring performance he was the pianist who played Tchaikovsky Piano Concerto No. 1.

Tchaikovsky Piano Concerto No. 1

After Russia was banned from all major sporting competitions from 2021 to 2023 by the World Anti-Doping Agency as a result of a doping scandal, those cleared to compete were allowed to represent the Russian Olympic Committee or Russian Paralympic Committee at the 2020 Summer Olympics and Paralympics and at the 2022 Winter Olympics and Paralympics. Instead of the national anthem of Russia, a fragment of Tchaikovsky Piano Concerto No. 1 was played as the "Anthem of Team".

YouTube Recording

Ben watched the 2022 Winter Olympics at his grandmother home and played Tchaikovsky Piano Concerto No. 1 on her grand piano. It was the first time he touched the piano's amazing shinny key board since 2015. A video recording of that event was shown on YouTube which was watched by an estimated audience of 137 viewers of neighbors, family, friends along with other anonymous individuals.

Hashish

Ahmad became addicted to Hashish a potent type of marijuana at the age of 17 when his father worked as a computer engineer in Hamburg, Germany. He was introduced to it during a rave party organized by a secondary school friend. Ahmad was amazed by the calming effects of Hashish which allowed him to overcome his shyness and social awkwardness. As if it transformed him from an introvert to a popular and attractive young man. He could not imagine living without Hashish and when his parents returned back to the US, he shifted his daily use to marijuana.

Hearing Voices

In his second year of college, Ahmad began to hear voices of demons telling him that he is worthless and that he needs to jump of a bridge. The intensity of the voices prevented him from fulfilling the academic demands of college. He was assessed and diagnosed at age 21 with schizophrenia.

Overweight

Quitting marijuana use and treatment with antipsychotics led to the remission of the hallucinations. Ahmad continued to receive monthly injection of the antipsychotic medications for a year and half. He gained significant weight and felt drowsy and fatigued. He received social security disability due to his inability to work. His parents were reluctant to discontinue the treatment. Ahmad wanted to be alert and to lose weight.

Moving

Despite eating a healthy diet and exercising daily, Ahmad continued to gain extra weight. His father found a better paying job as a computer engineer in a different state. Ahmad new psychiatrist initiated a regular monitoring program whereby a psychiatric trained nurse will assess Ahmad condition on a weekly basis following the discontinuation of the monthly antipsychotic injection.

Doing Well

Sixth months passed without treatment with antipsychotic medications. Ahmed did not experience any recurrence of hallucinations and did not use any marijuana. He enrolled in college to study and to follow his father footsteps and eventually become a computer engineer. He is maintaining an ideal body weight, eating healthy food and regularly exercising.

Unknown

It remains unclear if both Ben and Ahmad would have developed schizophrenia even if they have not used marijuana. Many research studies have concluded that marijuana use could trigger schizophrenia and other psychotic disorders in susceptible individuals. These individuals could also develop schizophrenia in their early adulthood if exposed to psychosocial and interpersonal stressors. Additionally many patients who developed schizophrenia due to marijuana use continued to exhibit psychotic symptoms even after stopping marijuana use.

What Is Known

The causes of schizophrenia are still unknown. The use of marijuana* may be a contributory factor in the development of schizophrenia, potentially increasing the risk of the disease in those who are already at risk. Marijuana use has also been associated with doubling the rate of schizophrenia.

Heed the Warning

No matter what causes schizophrenia Ben and Ahmad amazing recovery and their pursue of a productive life is a testimony, a silver lining, a reminder and a warning about the dire consequences of using marijuana. May we all heed that warning and spread that message to all who glibly use marijuana since its use has been legalized in 23 states, three U. S. territories, and Washington D. C. and in many countries across the globe.

* Hjorthøj C, et al. Association between cannabis use disorder and schizophrenia stronger in young males than in females. Psychological Medicine. DOI: 10. 1017/S0033291723000880 (2023).

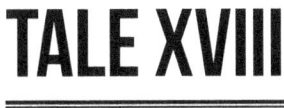

TALE XVIII

*Capgras Syndrome**
She Is Not My Wife

Capgras delusion or Capgras syndrome is a psychiatric disorder in which a person holds a delusion that a friend, spouse, parent, another close family member, or pet has been replaced by an identical impostor. It is named after Joseph Capgras, the French psychiatrist who first described the disorder.

Honeymoon Hotel

Zachary, a 73 year old gentleman was visiting the hotel where he had spent his honeymoon fifty years earlier. Since that visit he began referring to his wife as being her twin sister although there is no such person. In the meantime he accused his wife of being a liar and a cheat! His wife Sheila recalled that following their honeymoon Zachary cut all ties with his twin sister Coney due to her adamant opposition to their marriage. He would also frequently refer to Coney as being an "alien"! The conflict resolved when Coney dated one of Zachary's close friends and eventually she approved of his marriage to Sheila.

An Imposter

Zachary expressed feelings of intense anxiety related to fears that the wife's imposter will take advantage of his sound sleep and would poison him with carbon monoxide. He threatened to leave the home and to live in a shelter of the homeless. In response, Sheila suggested that she could move to reside with their younger son, while their older son come to stay with Zachary. He accepted the suggestion and expressed no more fears of being poisoned during his sleep. He continued to refer to Sheila as being an imposter and that she was not his wife but his wife's twin sister.

Delusion of Misidentification

Zachary's wife, his two sons and his twin sister Coney were quite concerned about his wellbeing. He agreed to be evaluated by his primary care physician Dr. Nolen. His medical evaluation revealed no medical or neurological problems that could cause the misidentification about his wife. Dr. Nolen diagnosed him with a delusional disorder and referred him for a psychiatric evaluation.

Capgras Syndrome

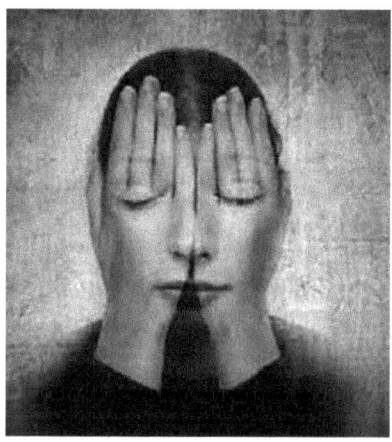

Despite his reluctance, Zachary undergone a psychiatric evaluation and was diagnosed with delusion of misidentification or Capgras syndrome. The recommendation was to use the antipsychotic medication haloperidol to reverse the delusion. Zachary refused to take the haloperidol and issued an ultimatum to his family "they either leave him alone along with the imposter wife or he will file a restraining order against them all".

A Psychoanalyst

Zachary twin sister Coney and her husband Eric every Summer rented a vacation home which they shared with another couple Rudolf and Josephine. Dr. Rudolf was a retired psychoanalyst who offered to assist Zachary's family. To the astonishment of everybody, Zachary agreed to meet Dr. Rudolf. He chose to meet him at the local golf club in one of their conference room. During their first meeting Dr. Rudolf introduced himself as an old-fashioned shrink!

An old-fashioned Shrink

Zachary could not stop laughing when he heard that introductory comment. He then asked about the purpose of their meeting. Dr. Rudolf paused, then answered if he wanted to find the whereabouts of Sheila his missing wife. Zachary then burst into tears and described how he was hurt and saddened by his twin sister Coney 's rejection of his marriage. He then described in details the reliving of these sad feelings during his recent stay in the same hotel where he had his honeymoon 50 years earlier.

Splitting of Thoughts

In their second meeting, Dr. Rudolf then clarified that it is possible that Zachary had to experience a splitting in his thinking. When splitting, the mind would accept and admire the good individual, the "real" person his wife Sheila, and reject the bad individual, the "imposter" or the "double", the wife's twin sister to be criticized and hated. The misidentification denies the authenticity and the identity of the person despite the admission of their apparent resemblances.

Torn by Love

Dr. Rudolf than proceeded to tell Zachary, that because he loved his twin sister Coney and also loved his bride Sheila, his mind had to split and unconsciously reject the notion that he had a twin sister, because that sister does not like his wife, so the fear of losing his wife created this delusion that most probably his wife Sheila is safer somewhere else, and the lady that lives with him is not his wife, but his wife's twin sister an imposter. By splitting he avoided having a conflict with his twin sister Coney. In reality Sheila was an only child and did not have any siblings.

She is my Wife

Zachary appeared to be relieved and he announced that he does miss his wife Sheila. Dr. Rudolf invited Sheila to join their meeting. Astonishingly, Zachary recognized her and wondered about why he has not seen her for a long time. He then asked if his twin sister Coney are still resentful and rejecting their marriage since they returned back from the hotel where they just spent their honeymoon. Sheila then clarified that their honeymoon was 50 years ago and at that time Coney his twin sister was not accepting their marriage and probably their recent stay in the same hotel could have triggered this episode of misidentification.

Re-experiencing

Dr. Rudolf then explained that the episode of misidentification and thinking that Sheila's twin sister who never existed was his wife imposter and an intruder is called Capgras syndrome and usually happened as a result of medical and neurological conditions. Since Zachary did not have any conditions to cause Capgras syndrome, most probably he developed it due to a psychological conflict. In that case, the conflict was Zachary's twin sister Coney, rejecting his wife Sheila. Although that conflict was resolved, it was re-experienced as a result of the recent stay in the same hotel, where Zachary and Coney spent their honeymoon.

The Trigger

Although psychoanalytic interpretation is not commonly included in today's clinical practice of psychiatry. Dr. Rudolf interpretation of Zachary's onset of Capgras syndrome was instrumental in the remission of his delusion of misidentification. The delusion was a firm belief that the person who described herself as his wife was rejected and addressed as an intruder, an imposter and as being his wife's Sheila twin sister who does not exist. . The interpretation also clarified the triggers that led to the re-experiencing of Zachary's twin sister Coney initial rejection of his marriage to Sheila during their honeymoon which was spent in the same hotel where Zachary and Sheila stayed recently.

Remember Psychoanalysis

Capgras syndrome with delusion of misidentification is usually a manifestation of medical or neurological conditions. It usually resolve once the underlying medical factors are diagnosed and treated. In today's hectic and busy psychiatric practices, there is not enough time to consider a psychoanalytic interpretation of presenting symptoms. It has been refreshing and inspiring to recognize Capgras syndrome that developed from psychological rather than medical factors.

Renewed Friendships

Zachary and his wife Sheila are thankful for the resolution of Capgras syndrome and they are close friends with Coney, Zachary's twin sister and her husband Eric. On special occasions they invited Dr. Rudolf and his wife Josephine to share in their Thanksgiving and Christmas celebrations

* Segments previously published in; Khouzam HR. Capgras Syndrome Responding to the Antidepressant Mirtazapine Comprehensive Therapy, 28(3):238-240, 2002.

TALE XIX

*Crisis Intervention**
A Public Health Prospective

A psychiatric emergency was called. A patient on the fourth hospital floor had found an unlocked window. He opened it and step out to stand on its exterior window edge. He threatened to jump off and crash to the ground. He wanted the whole world to know that he was mistreated by one of the hospital staff. He wanted the hospital to be closed and all its staff fired and punished for causing his death.

Difficult Hurdle

The psychiatric emergency team arrived on the scene. The fire department was called to install a life net to catch the patient if he jumps. The fears of his jumping prior to the arrival of the fire trucks imposed a difficult hurdle for the psychiatry emergency team. Any sudden approach to grab the patient's hand to prevent his jump could also jeopardize the team member who would attempt to do so.

What Do these Titles Mean?

I introduced myself to the patient as being the psychiatrist member of he emergency team. The patient shows signs of exasperation. He shouted a psychiatrist is not a "real doctor". I showed him my name tag with the title M.D. He said I doubted it, do you mean to tell me you are a psychiatrist and an M.D., I gently repeated a psychiatrist is an M.D. He maintained his balance to avoid falling and scratched his head and said and what is this other title next to M.D. ; M. P. H.

Prevention Types

He pronounced M.P.H. mpche. Are you also a veterinary, pal! I do not need the help of a doctor that treat pets and he leaned backward, stirring a panic in all the staff who were observing the scene, as he could have fallen from the window exterior edge. M. P. H. is a title that refer to Master of Public Health and not a veterinary doctor. What is that mean?. I clarified in public health for instance there is a concept of Primary Prevention, Secondary Prevention and Tertiary Prevention.

Frank is his Name

He seemed to be interested. I used his moment of silence to ask him. What is your name, Sir? I am no Sir, I am plain and simple Franklin Johnson. You can call me Frank, no fancy Sir, or Mr, got it? What is this Primary Prevention ? I gave an example of using the seat belt while driving to prevent serious injury in case of a car accident. He seemed to like this explanation and moved his right foot inside the window frame, while his left foot was still on the window exterior edge.

A Need for an Answer

Frank then proceeded to say, so Secondary Prevention is having 2 seat belts and Tertiary Prevention is having 3 seat belts and so on. Is that right doc?. Not knowing how to respond my mind wondered. If I remained silent, he may interpret it as belittling of his comments. If I respond, he may react negatively to my comments, causing further aggravation of his anger toward the hospital and its staff.

Whip Lash Complications

I responded by saying ;Mr. Johnson, although you asked me to address you as Frank, professionally I will call you using your last name. Ok he answered with some irritation. He then asked if he accurately explained Secondary Prevention and I asked if I could use the seat belt example. He nodded with an agreement gesture. If a person was using a seat belt then during a car accident experienced a whip lash, the Secondary Prevention would be to implement immediate therapeutic intervention to prevent possible complications of a whip lash. That person then did not receive any therapeutic intervention for his whip lash, then he could develop tendons, ligaments or neck bone fractures. Tertiary Prevention would then involve the prompt treatment of these injuries to avoid long term consequences of delaying such treatment which could lead to a permanent disability.

Half Way to Safety

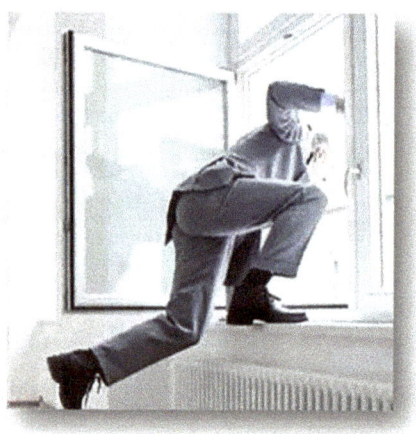

Mr. Johnson then moved his right foot from the window exterior edge to the inside of the window frame. He then gripped my hand and landed to the safety of the ground. He shook my hand and said "I am permanently disable" due to arthritis and earlier a receptionist was upset because I grabbed a wheelchair to sit while waiting for my name to be called. That made me angry and discouraged. I thought that by jumping out the window I would teach everybody in this hospital a lesson that will never forget. See Doc it would be a Primary Prevention to prevent the mistreatment of other patients.

Sigh of Relief

The hospital staff and the psychiatric emergency team that where witnessing the unfolding event expressed a sigh of relief. The fire department trucks did not install the life net. The eminent risk of jumping off the window was dissipated. Indescribable peace reigned and a life threatening crisis was avoided. Seeing Mr. Johnson voluntarily walking away from the window evoked spontaneous applauds from all who witnessed the potential of a disproportioned human tragedy.

A Reprimand

The next day I received a reprimand from my immediate supervisor and a harsh criticism from not following the safety protocols that prohibit grabbing the hand of a person who is attempting to jump from a building. These protocols precisely described the inherent risk of the rescuer being pulled by the person who is determined to jump resulting in a fatal crash of both individuals. My explanation of the fact that Mr. Johnson voluntarily walked away from the window to shake my hand did not achieve any success in withdrawing the reprimand.

Policy Over Hall

Mr. Johnson abandoned the idea of ending his life as a drastic measure to criticize the hospital and its staff. Instead he volunteered and joined the hospital 's department of public relations and wrote a summary detailing the dire consequences of ignoring patients with invisible disabilities such as arthritis. His writing had a far reaching effects and led to an overhaul of the hospital guidelines and policies that govern customer services and curtsey toward all patients including those with invisible disabilities.

Responding to the Moment

I was left to wonder about various other scenarios that could have helped resolved this eminent crisis. I could not discover or discern any. In that unprecedent event following the protocol would meant allowing Mr. Johnson to jump out the widow and fall on life net that would have been displayed by the fire trucks. Any miscalculation or delay in the arrival of the fire trucks would have led to a fatal crash.

Price of Ignoring a Protocol

A pearl of wisdom emerged from that event. Although safety protocols need to be followed without any deviation, certain emergent crises would dictate ignoring these protocols. A hard learned and worthwhile lesson that cost its practitioner a reprimand and a harsh criticism but saved a life that could have ended in a spectacular and tragic crash.

> * Segments previously presented in Grand Round Teaching Conference. "Taking Crisis Out of Crises", Department of Psychiatry Teaching Conference. The University of Oklahoma Health Sciences Center. December 5, 1991.